Cancer Hacks

A Holistic Guide to Overcoming
your Fears and Healing Cancer

Plus a 7-Day Healing Cleanse

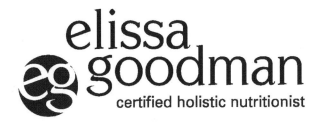

elissa
goodman
certified holistic nutritionist

Published by Best Seller Publishing®, Pasadena, CA
Best Seller Publishing® is a registered trademark
Printed in the United States of America.

ISBN-13: 978-1534741874
ISBN-10: 1534741879

MEDICAL DISCLAIMER:

This publication is designed to provide accurate and authoritative information with regard to the subject matter covered. It is sold with the understanding that the publisher is not engaged in rendering legal, accounting, or other professional advice. If legal advice or other expert assistance is required, the services of a competent professional should be sought. The opinions expressed by the authors in this book are not endorsed by Best Seller Publishing® and are the sole responsibility of the author rendering the opinion.

Most Best Seller Publishing® titles are available at special quantity discounts for bulk purchases for sales promotions, premiums, fundraising, and educational use. Special versions or book excerpts can also be created to fit specific needs.

For more information, please write:

Best Seller Publishing®
1346 Walnut Street, #205
Pasadena, CA 91106
or call 1(626) 765 9750
Toll Free: 1(844) 850-3500
Visit us online at: www.BestSellerPublishing.org

This book is dedicated with everlasting love and gratitude to all of my angels, without whom I could have survived the darkest times of my life:

My husband, Marc, who gave me a tremendous amount of love and laughs during the years we were together; My two daughters, Jordan and Samantha, who are both my constant source of strength and teach me important life's lessons every day; My mother and father, Karl and Stevie, who taught me to be resourceful and never give up; My fiancé, David, a treasure who came into my life at the right time and the right place; Alessandro, who taught me to find my voice and conquer all of my fears; Ryan, who had the inspiration for the book; Nora, who kept me motivated when I wanted to give up; Amber, who kept my business running without a hitch.

There are so many friends to thank that have been a constant and loyal support. You will know who you are when the book comes out, because I will be sending you a special note to say thank you!

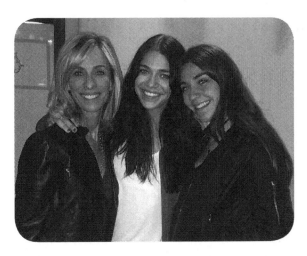

Contents

Introduction

If you are reading this book, it might be because you were just diagnosed with cancer, or you are in remission, or maybe someone you love has cancer, or maybe you are scared you are going to get cancer. If you are reading this book, chances are you do not know me personally; maybe you follow me on Instagram, Facebook, Pinterest, or Twitter; or have read my blog or participated in one of my Los Angeles cleanse programs.

Today, as I write this, I am 55 years old. I feel better than I have ever felt in my entire life. I have endured a cancer battle of my own, as well as losing my husband to cancer. I might not know you or your journey, but I know cancer and I know how significant my own journey with cancer was and is in my life.

Sometimes I wonder why I won my cancer battle but my husband did not. After decades of exploring this, I think it comes down to one major thing: at my core, instinctively, I knew I could and I would beat this. My husband, Marc, couldn't find the same confidence. He was frightened and only heard his doctors tell him he might not beat the disease.

I did not write this book to give you a list of ten things that you can do and then check off and then BAM! cancer is out of your life. That is unfortunately not how it works. There is no magic pill and there is not enough green juice in the world to wash away cancer. Which is scary and I get that.

I flew into a tailspin when I got diagnosed. It felt like I had been beaten down my whole life and this was just the culmination of all those beatings. It is not my personality to take charge and fix things. I like to be taken care of; I like to find experts and have them

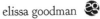
elissa goodman

tell me what to do. It is easier that way, right? And they must know the best plan if they are the experts, don't they?

I am here to tell you that the answer to those questions is NO. So, if I am the expert you are coming to, do not just take what I say as the only path to follow. I am here to be a guide, to share my emotional journey as well as the extensive research and my real-life experiences to help you in your battle with the wretched disease we've both faced. I hope some things in my book will speak to you, and I hope you will feel connected to some of the stories I share.

With that said, the thing I want you to take away from this book is that YOU are in control. And more than that, YOU have the ability to know how to heal. My clients and my kids can all tell you that if I preach anything, it's to trust your gut. Something in this book will hit home for you. Hopefully, it will be more than one thing. You will connect with what you need. Trust that—there is a reason that it's speaking to you. Cancer changed a lot of things in my life, but most significantly it empowered me to take care of me.

In the years I have spent since my own cancer diagnosis helping others in similar situations, it feels as though the cycle of healing has been completed. If you had told me, when I was 32, sitting in that doctor's office hearing that diagnosis and scared out of my mind, that I would not only overcome cancer, but one day would help others overcome it as well, I would have never believed you.

With this book, I extend the healing cycle to you. May you understand that everyone in your shoes has at one point felt alone, scared, and powerless. But may you learn that you are *not* alone; you *can* face your fears and *regain* your power. That is what these hacks are—ways to put you back in the driver's seat. Yes, something foreign and scary has taken over your body. But it is still *your* body and it is yours to be loved and cared for and healed.

Let's do it together.

My Cancer Journey

Today, I am at my happiest and healthiest but life has not always been that way. When I look back at my childhood, I am struck by all the memories I have of being sick. I had severe eczema, low red-blood-cell count, digestive and respiratory issues, mono, and consistent low energy. I felt like I could never catch a break.

When I meet with new clients, we start from the beginning. So I'm going to do the same with you. My dad was a successful businessman in Arizona and both my parents were extremely Type A. Every day they had a mile-long to-do list and by sundown everything had a check mark next to it. They were the most motivated and successful people I've ever witnessed and they both had endless energy. I used to think that when I grew up, I too would want to get up at 5 AM to exercise every morning. Turns out I didn't inherit that gene!

I lived in awe of everything they accomplished in a day; there was never a task too large or too few hours available. I was so impressed by them, but I could never match their energy or drive. I didn't know how to be the people they were; and I didn't know how to want the things they wanted. From an early age, I never felt like I was doing enough.

This feeling stayed with me throughout my childhood. I felt like I could not figure out my place in my own family. I felt like I was constantly treading water, trying to stay afloat, keep up, and make my parents proud. I was so different from them and their opinions were strong. No matter the subject, I was convinced I was wrong. In those days, the mentality of parents was that children should be "seen and not heard."

Not many families I knew encouraged kids to march to the beat of their own drummer; it was more about marching in line. In my house, there was one way that things were going to go and that was it; it did not matter if that did not feel right to me. I worked hard to be a good kid but I also started second-guessing everything and got consumed by self-doubt. I had a hard time trusting my inner voice, because I did not have the confidence to share it.

My dad had started from nothing and worked really, really hard. He and my mom deserved the life they built together and they tried to show me how to follow them on their path to success. But I was not the same as them and was never going to find success faking it. I fell into a bad pattern of questioning my worth and always trying to prove myself to others. It was not until recently that I realized you can take certain positive aspects from your parents and carry those with you—you don't have to become the exact person your parents were or are.

I am far from being the exact person either of them were at this age, but they are a part of me and I am beyond grateful for the things I have taken from them. My dad gifted me an incredible sense of drive, determination, and capacity to always see the glass as half full. My mom deserves a lot of credit for being the first person to expose me to a holistic and healthier lifestyle.

My mom suffered from asthma her entire life. In fact, that is the reason why she moved from a small town in Illinois to Tucson, Arizona, to go to college. The dry air and heat helped, but it never went away. In the 1970s, she discovered a health ranch in Tecate, Mexico, called Rancho La Puerta. She went twice a year for seven days and she would take a number of friends with her each time. When I was 15 years old she started including me.

This place was her sanctuary. She looked forward to going again the minute she got home. It was really ahead of its time. The ranch chefs grew their own food and we ate whole, nutrient-dense food at every meal. The women devoured and licked their plates clean. We exercised daily starting with a 6 AM hike to see the sun rise.

I would get major anxiety about this hike, because hiking did not come naturally to me and getting up at 5:30 surely was not my idea of fun. After the hike, I was ready for a nap, but there were so many exercise classes to choose from that I felt guilty not taking advantage of them.

Mom always dragged me to yoga, which I thought was boring. The meditation was painful, because it forced me to think about what was not working in my life. I remember thinking about all the things I needed to change when I got home, which I did not do. Mom also insisted on us getting a daily massage or facial. I was still shy about my body then, so being naked on a massage table when the masseuses barely covered you was embarrassing. Also, they would slap you around like a piece of meat. In those days, the mentality was the harder they massaged you, the better it was for your body, even bruises were a badge of honor.

By the middle of the week, I did notice I felt different and the women who were there were different people. It was incredible! They felt better, they were more energetic, they were happier, they were calmer, and some were thinking about lowering the dosages of their medication. Even Mom, who relied heavily on her asthma medication, seemed to not need it as much or as often!

Now, I would do anything to go back to that ranch every year and maybe twice a year too. But at the time, I would have done anything to leave. The idea that I had to sleep in the same room as my mom and only interact with adult women for seven days was terrifying. I wasn't ready for meditation, yoga, and healthy food. I wanted to be home with my friends, sitting on my butt watching TV, and going to eat whatever I wanted whenever I wanted it.

Also, there was only one phone at the ranch and you had to sign up to use it and it wasn't cheap. Mom always knew when I was calling my friends, so I couldn't do it often. Distractions didn't exist at the ranch, and I was forced to give in fully to the experience. The idea of getting in touch with myself was frightening. I was not ready to deal with the demons and anxieties that were inside me. I did not know how to handle my problems and my insecurities. I thought that running away was the only safe way to deal with things. But looking back at the experience, I can honestly say I felt my first sense of peace there.

I think that is why, as soon as I graduated from college, I left Arizona. I knew I needed the independence to try to get in touch with myself and find my drive and inner strength. I thought by getting away it would help me find my own pace and find a way of life that worked for me. But I went right to New York City and started working a fast-paced job. I was always really stressed, but I hid it with caffeine, alcohol, and some nights I would go home and eat a pint of Ben & Jerry's ice cream for dinner. It was my reward for surviving the day.

I had gone to New York City with my Arizona style—yes, that meant hair to match. I was working as an intern at a TV rep firm and my hairdo was definitely not sophisticated or city chic. A handsome sales rep, named Marc, kindly told me that I would never get a job with that 'do. Off to the salon I went! Thankfully, the hairdo left but the handsome sales rep stayed.

Marc reminded me a lot of my dad. He was incredibly motivated, determined to succeed, outgoing, and everyone loved him. We fell in love and it felt like I was living the New York City dream. Something about being in New York and working crazy hours and living independently from my parents really stoked the feeling that I could make them proud. Most days, fueled by coffee and bagels, I felt physically awful but I kept pushing. I romanticized my life there; I thought that this was just the ladder you had to climb to get your dream life.

Marc and I got married and joined our hectic lives together. Shortly after we were married, however, he got transferred to Los Angeles. Although we had built a fun and exciting life in New York, I remember feeling a total sense of relief. Los Angeles meant a new way of life; we could calm down, breathe, and start a family. I could finally find the peace I had been looking for my whole life.

Not long after being in LA, I was getting a massage when the masseuse felt a swollen lymph node on my collarbone. She suggested I get it checked out right away and I did. Sure enough, she had cause for her concern: I had cancer. Never before have I so appreciated a massage!

If you have been in that room, hearing, "you have cancer," you can appreciate the total sense of fear that takes over. I was 32 years old. My doctors were not even sure what kind of cancer it was, yet they wanted to start radiation treatments and chemotherapy immediately. There was a terrifying sense of urgency and panic; they told me I better freeze my eggs if I ever wanted to have kids. I get sick now thinking about how overwhelmed I was.

But there was that little voice inside me, the one that had been told to hide away my whole childhood, the one I ignored while I partied away at every happy hour in New York City. It was still with me and now, more than ever, it wasn't going to let me silence it.

You will get all the details in the rest of the book, but, long story short, I listened to my inner voice; I did things my way, with the doctor I chose and the path that made sense to me and my gut. I said no to the chemotherapy and freezing my eggs. I said no to the long, intensive radiation and agreed to doing a shorter regimen of localized radiation. I started therapy, yoga, and meditating. I started eating alkaline foods and juicing like crazy. At that time, you could not get a juice on every corner like you can today. I went to Beverly Hills Juice (which is still around and still a local favorite) where they had fairly limited options. I drank so much carrot juice my palms turned orange. But I didn't care. For the first time in my life, I felt like I was in control, taking charge and healing. Less than a year after my diagnosis, I was cancer free.

Calm was restored in my life, and Marc and I became the parents to two beautiful, healthy girls. But the storm wasn't over. Twelve years after my diagnosis, cancer hit us again. My Hodgkin's lymphoma was long gone, but Marc had just been diagnosed with Non-Hodgkin's lymphoma. It was truly hard to believe.

elissa goodman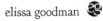

Marc fought his cancer in a different way than I did. He immediately began intense chemotherapy. He spent his 18-month battle in and out of the hospital. Part of the connection we felt early in our relationship was based on Marc's and my similar lack of self-worth. I think the cancer made him feel so terrified that if he didn't survive, it would show his weaknesses.

Marc's dad had died of cancer when Marc was two years old. His whole life, I think he carried this imprint that if you get cancer, you die. He was angry, and rightfully so. We had just settled into a calm, lovely life. He was at his dream job, the girls were great, and we had just remodeled a house we loved. It was really hard work to get to that place in life and now it felt like everything was crashing down again. He started to take on this blame as if it was his fault. He was scared that he couldn't fight his disease.

A year after he was diagnosed, his doctor told him he would probably die. He accepted this like it was fact—he was scared and he went into dying mode. He wanted comfort food, not healthy food. His doctors were against him taking any vitamins or supplements and he listened to them. His immune system was so badly weakened from the chemo, radiation, and bone marrow transplants that when infection struck him after he had fought for a year and half, his body gave in to it.

The greatest lesson I learned from losing Marc is that when you are sick, a lot of people think your battle has to be about finding something worth living for. I know Marc would have given everything he had to live for our daughters. But the truth is, you have to believe that you, *yourself*, are worth living for. What do YOU want out of this life? What can YOU offer the world? Marc was so terrified and could not see his own light at the end of the tunnel. I have been in those dark places too and to be able to climb out of them is like mentally climbing Mount Everest. But it is worth it.

After Marc died, I was left alone as a single, widowed mom with two heartbroken young girls. The idea that I was going to have to raise them alone was petrifying to me. I told myself I wasn't capable;

I did not feel like I had the skills. I relived the friction that I had in my relationship with my own mother and created the same discord with my daughters. I became my own worst nightmare: it was my way or the highway. I did not know how to really listen to their opinions and thoughts and desires and dreams; I wanted to protect them and I felt I had to control them.

My oldest daughter was the opposite of me. She was fearless and an old soul; she could sense all the turmoil I was going through and she wanted to talk about it. I wanted to shove it under the rug and just move on—that is how I always dealt with stuff. This did not sit well with her.

The three of us are so connected in such a deep way; it is scary and beautiful at the same time. It was really scary to have a 13 year old calling me out on my shit; she exposed my weaknesses.

Motherhood taught me the power of surrendering. My daughters are their own people, with their own paths. Who am I to say they cannot do something just because it is something I would not do? The greatest lesson I have ever learned is that you have to have faith in yourself, faith in your life, and faith that everything does work out. I had to have faith that my daughters could be themselves and still be okay. That I could let them do things their way sometimes and they would survive.

How could I teach them to trust themselves, if I did not give them the chance to make their own choices? Trust me, this isn't always easy (especially in their teenage years!) but I saw the stranglehold style of parenting was not working out. My daughters taught me how to let go of trying to control everything that scared me and instead to have faith.

I cherish the time I had with the girls, but there was still a traditional bug inside me that felt like I had to find a new husband. I still did not totally trust myself to raise these girls alone and I was in a rush to get remarried. I met a wonderful man named David and, for me, it was love at first sight and I was ready to settle down right away.

Luckily, David had a bit more sense of what was going on. He was recently divorced and didn't want to jump into getting married again. I think he also understood what was happening with me. Our love was real, but where I was in my life was confusing. David told me I needed to spend more time with me, to find my passion and purpose. He told me he could not be with me until I found myself.

Of course, I was heartbroken then, but now I realize it was one of the greatest gifts I ever received. It started an internal conversation within me that was much needed. I realized I had never had a job or career that I loved. I realized that every job and career I had up to that point was something that I thought I should have. It was a scary but invigorating moment—what would I do if I went back to square one?

I brought this up over lunch with a friend one day. She started asking me questions about what I was passionate about; prodding toward the things that I loved to do, seek, and learn. I realized that getting cancer was the first time I had really stepped up and taken control. I cared about the process and the results. I was fascinated by everything I learned in my experience as well as in watching Marc's experience. I realized that I wanted to help people who were going through what I had been through.

It felt like such a natural move, I had always been interested in nutrition, though I was not following it consistently myself. But I had dabbled in it and applied what I learned at the ranch with Mom to help me with different ailments through the years, such as digestion issues, sinus issues, and anxiety. I ended up signing up for a two-year holistic nutrition certification program at the University of Complementary Medicine in Beverly Hills. I fell in love with my classes and I felt so happy being in school. Before that, I had convinced myself that I wanted to get married again and have someone support me, but in my inner core I wanted to do things for myself and get back to the world. I was excited about life again.

One day, David called me out of the blue. He had suffered with a bad cough for a year, had gotten pneumonia, and had a bunch

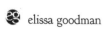 elissa goodman

of scans done. He was scared and convinced he might have lung cancer. He had to go in for a test where they were going to biopsy tissue out of his lungs and he wanted me to go with him. It felt like a light bulb had gone off for him that I could be someone to support him like he could support me. While we were apart, I had become independent, I was in school, and I was finding my way. What we could offer each other was love and support and it was mutual. We both needed it.

Thank God, he didn't have lung cancer, but he did radically change his diet to eliminate gluten, sugar, dairy, and alcohol. That last one definitely put a damper on our dinners or nights out with friends! But his cough went away and six months later it was gone permanently. Guess what? The only time it returns is when he is super stressed and he falls off the wagon with his food choices. Helping him made me feel destined to help others in this way. It gave me purpose and gave me proof that food and the way you treat your body does make a huge difference.

When I graduated from school, I was fortunate to have a friend give me the opportunity to create a cleanse program for the newest, hottest vegan restaurant in Los Angeles, called Cafe Gratitude. I was panicked and did not feel capable, but I said yes. I poured myself into research about cleansing and what that meant. It's been mostly about juice cleanses that have no food and this didn't sit right with me so I went back to the books.

One day, something clicked. The life I lived and the foods I ate were cleansing. I drank juice, but I also ate, whole, nutrient-dense foods. I was experiencing great results without all the deprivation or starvation. And I could do it every day—not just for a limited period of time.

I created this alternative cleanse with more of a lifestyle mentality. It was a huge hit and put me on the map. Also, cleansers had the option to have me help them with any health concerns. This was before I had my own clients and I learned so, so much. It was one of the greatest experiences of my life. I got to talk to all these

 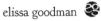

different people, with all these different ailments. I call this time my "residency" as I was thrown into the deep end a bit and had to do a lot of work to help these people. It could not have been a better experience.

Six months later, I got a call from the owner of another huge macrobiotic health spot in LA, called M Cafe. He had seen my cleanse program and wanted me to develop a program for his restaurant as well. I was in heaven!

Both of these programs led me to having private clients of my own. I used to be scared to meet with people one-on-one. My old insecurities came out and told me that I would not survive if I couldn't reach for a book or search for something online. But client after client, I realized I did have the tools and the knowledge but, most of all, I had the experience. I wasn't some expert telling these people how to live their lives; I was their equal. I had walked in their shoes. We could share our experiences with each other.

This quickly became the favorite part of my business; it is truly the best feeling in the world. There is something about that intimate connection with people and, most important, being able to give them hope. I once had a friend comment that once I had enough success I wouldn't have to see personal clients anymore. I told her she was crazy! I would never give that part of my business up. It's the reason I'm here, the reason I feel so emotionally tied to what I do, and the reason I get up every morning. I've found my passion!

In the few years since all this began, I have been more than blessed with amazing opportunities. I've been able to help hundreds of clients, I created an online 21-day do-it-yourself cleanse program called, "Cleanse Your Body, Cleanse Your Life", and a home-cooked 5-day S.O.U.P. Cleanse that I deliver locally. I've even gotten to design juices for Erewhon Natural Health Market and LA Juice. I recently designed a whole new menu for Earth Bar, a longtime favorite juice, smoothie, and supplement place with 22 locations.

I built a beautiful life with my two girls, David, and his two sons. The kids don't always love having a nutritionist pick what's for dinner, but they are making strides. I try to remember how resistant I was at the ranch with my mom. I learned that I cannot tell them what to do and I cannot be there for every meal checking for gluten, sugar, or anything heavily processed.

You can give your kids tools. Tools to make the right decisions and to trust their own instincts. Tools to take care of themselves when you cannot be there. I want my kids to have the tools to feel good, to have purpose, and to have the inner strength I never thought I had.

Now, I appreciate and soak up the moments when my youngest daughter asks for a green juice or my oldest daughter sends a picture of the wild-caught salmon and veggies she made for dinner. They have tools to ask for and seek what's good for them and that is something I'm very proud of.

One of my favorite books is *The Alchemist* by Paulo Coelho. The main character kept having to face obstacle after obstacle, but he had a strong inner core that told him he could survive. I feel that way about myself. Even in my lowest moments, I feel like I can survive. When I had cancer, often I did not know what to do, but I had enough to push myself forward and figure out the "how" along the way. The obstacles presented to the character in the Coelho book always offered a lesson and equipped him with the wisdom and skill to use against his next obstacle. Oh, can I relate!

Before I used to think I just had bad karma, now I feel lucky for the lessons—I think to myself, bring them on! Things go wrong and I truly think "thank God, I can learn something new." That did not happen until my 50s. I never thought I would be secure in myself or be a calm mother. I never thought I would really respect other people's opinions, especially my kids. I found out, "my way or the highway" is an isolating, lonely, unhealthy life.

I would like to help people embrace the lessons a little earlier and tap into the confident, optimistic voice I know we all have deep down. The voice that tells us that we are worth it, our lives are worth it, and fighting for our lives is worth it.

I am so lucky to be able to do what I do. Not a day goes by that I don't feel overwhelmed with gratitude and thanks for all the people who supported me along the way. But I also feel like fate had a role in where I am today. I spent my life being sick or scared or mourning my losses. But here I am, finally having experienced the light at the end of the tunnel. And I want you to know, that there's light for you too. So let's get moving and get you there.

Cancer Myths

Cancer

Say that out loud a few times. Pay attention to how it feels in your body to say and acknowledge that word. Do you feel your throat tightening around it? Does it evoke feelings of fear and uncertainty?

Cancer is terrifying. It's the unknown, it's malevolent, and it's confusing. Chances are you know at least a few people touched by cancer. You might have even lost a family member or a friend to cancer. Within the United States, cancer is the number one health concern. It's a growing epidemic and it can feel like a monstrous power that is taking over our world.

When confusion strikes, fear sets in, and fear can lead us to cling to information, just for the simple fact that it is information. It is important for you to understand that there is so much evidence that what we believe to be true about cancer is wrong. And many universal truths we think we know about cancer do not apply to everyone with cancer.

I want you to take a deep breath and let go of the feelings you felt when you said the word cancer. It's just a word. And you are a human who is powerful and strong and able to educate yourself on what that word really means.

Let's break down some cancer myths.

Myth #1:
What You Put in Your Body
Doesn't Cause Cancer

The world's largest ongoing analysis of diet and cancer research shows that at least one third of the most common cancers could be prevented if we ate a healthy diet. In my world, a healthy diet is following the 80/20 plan. For example, 80 percent of the time, I eat clean, whole, nutrient-dense foods. But listen, no nutritionist in the world eats that clean all the time and if they tell you they are, they are lying to you. And 20 percent of the time, I allow myself to indulge in moderation.

Throughout the course of this book, I am going to detail what I recommend you eat 80 percent of the time. I won't spend much time talking about the 20 percent but, just so you know, for me, it's dark chocolate, tequila, wine, In-N-Out Burgers, and extra crispy potato chips.

If clients show up on my doorstep, they have some awareness that their diet needs help. That is why they see a nutritionist, right? Often times, my clients have tried to get healthy on their own. They have bought cookbooks, read blogs, and taken supplements, but they still hit a roadblock.

Here is the thing about eating healthy: it could not be simpler. But changing your lifestyle can feel foreign and scary. What do you snack on if for the past five years you have snacked on 100-calorie packs? What do you make for dinner if I tell you to throw away every Lean Cuisine in your freezer?

For a lot of you, eating the way I describe in this book means breaking out of your comfort zone in a big way. I want you to be comfortable. So, I'm going to let you in on a little secret. I read a lot of blogs like my own that share tons of amazing healthy recipes. Recipes that would blow any meat-and-potatoes guy out of the

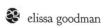 elissa goodman

water. I'm going to be honest with you—when I share a recipe, I share it because it is delicious but also because it is unique, special, and interesting. Nobody wants to see a recipe of my go-to avocado smeared on gluten-free bread on my blog every week. And, no one is begging for the recipe of leftover quinoa thrown together with the spinach I sautéed because it was about to go bad.

So, if you are sitting there, wondering how you will ever have the time or the energy to eat this way or if you are looking online to determine what a spiralizer is, relax. I am a working mother with tons of interests and hobbies and activities. I do not spiralize every meal I make. I prepare, I plan, and I do my best. And sometimes I eat gluten-free toast smeared with avocado every day for a week.

Initially, there might be some work you have to do, and preparation is going to make your life a lot easier, but eating healthy takes the same amount of effort as eating crappy. You are still going to the grocery store and picking out what to eat. Now you are going to spend your time in the produce department, not in the cookie aisle. You are still going to go out to eat with your friends. You are just going to choose a healthier option than a big bowl of Fettuccine Alfredo or a steak and fries.

And here is my promise to you—eating this way will not *take* more energy, but it will *give* you more energy. My clients always start out by dreading spending the time to chop veggies, but within a week or two they call me to say that they have never accomplished more in a day in their lives.

You will be flooded with information in the rest of the book, but right now I want to show you that eating this way is not that intimidating. My basic rules for eating clean are to eat whole, real foods; radically reduce your sugar consumption; limit your animal protein, caffeine, and alcohol consumption; and be smart when you eat out. I mentioned my 80/20 rule. It's truly as simple as that. At least 80 percent of the time, your diet should be whole foods and not processed. As a culture, we need to open our eyes to all the chemicals in our food. We have to stop assuming that the stuff being

elissa goodman

sold to us is okay to consume. We have to pay attention. The faker our food industry gets, the more disease levels skyrocket. When are we going to acknowledge a connection? We need to wake up and use our common sense and recognize that this is not working.

The lifestyle plan I preach does not mean you can never splurge again; it just means that you provide your body with the best nutrients for it most of the time so that it can still thrive despite those Margarita and chip indulgences. Cleaning up your diet does not need to be a complicated process. Load up on whole, real foods, meaning fruits, veggies, legumes, whole grains (preferably gluten-free, such as quinoa, brown rice, and millet), organic, non-processed meats, fish, and tofu. It means limiting dairy and gluten, which are often extremely processed. It means not overdoing it on animal protein, not downing a bottle of wine every night, and not letting a pitcher of Margaritas and a bowl of salty chips send you into full-on binge mode. It means what you eat should not have a shelf-life or an ingredient you cannot pronounce. No, French fries are not a whole food; yes, potatoes are.

Forget what all those years of fad diets have told you. Ignore the people who tell you this way of eating is a fad diet. This way of eating is getting back to basics, back before preventable disease ravaged our country because of what we put in our bodies. Sugar has proven time and again to feed cancer. Many years ago, food companies tapped into the incredibly marketable and hypnotizing way that our bodies respond to sugar. Sugar is one of the most addictive substances known to humankind. In a study in which rats were given the choice between sugar water and cocaine, 94 percent of the time, they chose the sugar water. Then the researchers studied rats who were already addicted to cocaine. Even those rats chose sugar water over cocaine when given the choice. This is extremely alarming!

While following the 80/20 plan, the best advice I can give you is to take the 20 percent and spread it around. So many people now do "cheat days" or "cheat meals." Little splurges throughout the week allow you to never feel like you are holding back. Wasting your 20 percent on a whole day or one huge meal is setting yourself up for failure, it puts so much pressure on the rest of the week that you will buckle.

But also, never forget, tomorrow is a new day. You can drive yourself crazy over what you ate or you can learn a lesson and start fresh tomorrow.

Myth #2:
Cancer Is a Death Sentence

The word "cancer" carries so much weight but the diagnosis does not always match it. Cancer is no longer the automatic death sentence it was once feared to be. Millions and millions of people survive cancer every year.

One of the tricky things with getting a cancer diagnosis is that the liability for doctors has grown so immensely in the past few years. Often, in protection of their own selves, they are setting you up for the worst-case scenario. They are worried you will eventually get a cancer diagnosis that they did not catch and come back and sue them. If a doctor says you have cancer, you should listen, but you should also get multiple opinions and do your own research. Taking on the mentality that your worst-case scenario is your reality can be lethal.

Our minds are so powerful; you have to be careful what you allow them to believe.

We allow fear to set us in our ways. If you know someone who died from cancer, you take on the fear and the idea that if you get cancer it is or could be a death sentence. We see it a lot with breast cancer. Today, women who have breast cancer in their family get a double mastectomy before any cancer is ever detected.

In my opinion, that is quite radical. It is the quick-fix culture we seek. We think, "If my breasts are gone, I cannot get breast cancer," but you cannot just chop off parts of your body out of fear. Preventive measures, like getting regular checkups paired with living the cancer-fighting lifestyle I talk about in this book, are the best way to handle the fear of getting cancer.

You might have a gene that passes cancer through your family, but that gene has to be activated by lifestyle choices. We make such rash decisions out of fear and put so much focus on what we think is inevitable. Think about it—the first thing a doctor does is ask you for the medical history of your parents and grandparents. I'm not trying to diminish the fact that this plays a role, but we cannot put all our thoughts into a potential predisposition. Just because your mother died from cancer does not mean you will. My belief system is that anything can be changed. You have a different genetic makeup and a different life than your parents or grandparents. Anything can be prevented.

We need to stop running to the solution before the problem shows itself. And we need to stop believing that if the problem shows itself, that it has the same outcome as other people's cancer stories. Your story is unique and it can go any way you want it to. Prevention, getting to know your body, and distinguishing between fear and gut instinct are the best ways to handle a fear of cancer.

One of my main reasons for writing this book is that I want people to know that cancer does not mean death. It wasn't that long ago that pneumonia meant death. Things change, we evolve. Cancer today does not mean what it meant even five or ten years ago. Today, we have more tools than ever to combat this disease and your chances of surviving are higher than ever.

Myth #3:
Cancer Is Contagious

Similar to those who are sure they will get cancer because their parents had it, there are many who think they can get cancer from other people. If you inherit a cancerous gene, you will still have to set it off with lifestyle choices. Similarly, if you get a cancer-causing virus, such as hepatitis B, helicobacter pylori (H pylori), or human papillomavirus (HPV) from someone, you would have to provoke it with lifestyle choices. All of these infections can lay dormant within you if you take cancer-fighting precautions. Some infections, like human immunodeficiency virus (HIV), can suppress your immune system, making your body a welcoming home for cancer. So you have to boost your immunity and make sure you are taking extra precautions to avoid letting cancer pounce on a precious immune system.

In my world, everyone has cancer. I know that can be scary to think about but it also gives you the power to not entice it to come out and play. Cancer is not something you catch from the world, it is something that was within you, and somewhere along the way, diet, habits, lack of exercise, emotional baggage, stress, trauma, or likely some combination lured it to come out and show itself.

Stop fearing that you can get cancer from someone else. Instead go hug someone with cancer. It is proven that a hug can send you into relaxation mode, which is where healing happens. How cool is that—you will not get cancer from them, but you might help take it away.

Myth #4:
One Mistake Can Cause Cancer

Almost as often as I see clients come in who have no clue as to what caused their cancer, I have clients come in who are so sure what did

 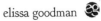

cause it. They are positive it was all the cigarettes they smoked, or their relationship with their father, or the fact that they have never tried Brussels sprouts.

Listen, I know that I have written a whole book about things that can play into cancer, but I need you to know that there are SO many things at play. Putting the blame on one item is not helpful or healthy. You cannot heal if you are focused on one regret. Instead of heckling yourself for smoking so many cigarettes, ask yourself what you can do in your whole life to make yourself healthier. You cannot make progress unless you take responsibility for all the areas in your life that are unhealthy. People smoke a pack a day and drink every night and can live into their 90s. Cause and effect with cancer is not black and white.

We are always looking for a "why," because we want an answer and a cause. I am here to tell you that, unfortunately, even if you have a really good idea, you will not ever really know why things happen the way they do. That is unsettling, I know. But it is life and you can drive yourself crazy trying to figure out why. Let's not focus on the past—let's focus on the future. How can you make yourself become a cancer-fighting machine today?

Myth #5:
Stress Doesn't Cause Cancer

This is a biggie for me and in our world, it is so important. Scientists have discovered that everyday emotional stress is a trigger for tumor growth. Any sort of emotional or physical trauma can act as a pathway between cancerous cell mutations. These findings show that the conditions for developing cancer can be affected by your everyday work and family stress.

Until now, scientists believed more than one cancer-causing mutation needed to take place in a single cell in order for tumors to grow. However, researchers showed that mutations could promote cancer even when they are located in different cells, because stress opens up "pathways" between them. I have long believed that emotional factors are one of the most important contributing factors for all diseases, especially cancer and the studies are showing that is true.

You do not have to be the president of the United States or a CEO of a huge company to be stressed. Our environment is grooming us to be constantly stressed. The line at Starbucks is stressful, the traffic on the way to work is stressful, what you are going to wear to your sister's wedding is stressful, and how the kids are going to get to their piano lessons is stressful. Our current culture is stressed and it is causing cancer to host a party in our bodies. We are driven and anxious and have such a desire to keep up with this crazy fast culture and environment and it is making us sick.

Ever since I met Marc, he was always stressing about something. He did not know how to live any differently and most certainly did not think he would get cancer from it. This way of life was getting him ahead in his career, his golf game, and his social circle. When Marc was diagnosed, he continued his stressful way of doing things. He never gave himself a break. Our bodies cannot heal while we are stressed and we become our own worst enemies.

Marc and I were evenly matched in this area of our lives, but because of my time at Rancho La Puerta, I knew how important it is to de-stress to heal and be healthy. In this book, I will share with you some of those ways to de-stress in simple, easy, and effective ways. Stress and anxiety are the products of fear and fear is not having faith. If you are stressed, deep down you worry about the future. We don't always have the confidence that everything will be okay. More than that, we need to be okay with not being okay. That's a huge step for cancer fighters. You are not okay, but you can be and you will be.

You cannot just eat kale, meditate, exercise, and stop drinking. You have to manage your stress. I think this is so important. I am not a huge fan of prescription drugs. I think we are overmedicated and constantly avoiding the root issue. But sometimes we need

 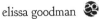

medicine to manage our stress and anxiety so that we can get to a place where we can take care of ourselves.

There are lots of fabulous herbal anti-anxiety options but if you need something stronger, ask for it. This is such a huge, huge, huge part of kicking cancer to the curb. If you sit in meditation but your mind cannot stop churning, you cannot reap the benefits of meditating. You need to get your head on straight so that you can calmly and proactively take care of yourself. You can always light up a joint. This might make you laugh, but marijuana does wonders for those dealing with stress. And, hey, I said whatever it takes. ☺

I started my blog because I saw how many misconceptions there were about cancer in today's world. It's never too late to take control of your life. Even if you don't have a diagnosis, it's never too late to reduce your risk. There's so much information flying around in the world that we are desperate to listen to anyone who speaks to us with authority. You have the authority over your body and the choices you make in your life. Forget everything you thought you knew about cancer. Start believing in this statement:

"I have the power and ability to take control, heal my cancer, and heal my life."

HACK 1:
The Standard American Diet

Did you know the FDA doesn't know about the safety and identity of an estimated 1,000 chemicals in our food because companies do not disclose them?

—Maricel V. Maffini, PhD, Natural Resources Defense Council, April 2014

Did you know more than 3,000 food additives—preservatives, flavorings, colors, and other ingredients—are added to US foods?

—Dr. Joseph Mercola, Mercola.com, February 2013

Did you know the European Union has banned all hormones in beef and Japan, Canada, Australia, New Zealand, and the EU have banned rBGH, the hormone that increases the amount of milk dairy cows produce?

—WebMD, 2013

I once had a new client come in, and immediately after I opened the door, I could tell she didn't want to be here. It was like she came in with a grudge, even though this was the first time we had met. Another client, who I adored, referred her so I was not sure what was happening. We started talking about her diet and it was so difficult. She knew what to eat—she barely touched carbs, she never ate candy, and salads were her go-to. She still did not feel healthy and that is why she was in my office.

In so many ways, I understood her frustration. She was a smart and health-conscious woman and she felt like she should have all the

 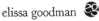

answers already, so why did she have to pay me her hard-earned money so that I could tell her how to eat healthy?

We dug a bit deeper into her diet. She "steered clear of sweets," yet she ate a processed chocolate brownie protein bar almost every morning. She had swapped her morning coffee for tea, but she still put a heavily processed salad dressing on all her salads. Her vegetable intake was incredible, but there was no balance— she rarely ate fruit, gluten-free grains, or healthy fats. And she was loading up on protein, eating animal protein three times a day. Among her seemingly healthy lifestyle, she had acquired some really bad habits, influenced by our dramatically changing food world, where being healthy for major food companies became all about fewer calories and cheap ingredients.

I totally felt for her as I had been in her shoes. I spent years of my life feeling like I was fairly healthy—at least healthier than a lot of the people around me. I never ate what people consider "junk food," I didn't smoke cigarettes, and I was not overweight. I grew up in a family where we were educated about nutrition and I had always been interested in it, so I made a point to keep educating myself.

But it's a really hard thing when rich, intelligent marketers are selling you something as "healthy" to know that it is incorrect. It is a really hard thing when you are trying to look and feel your best to not listen when someone says you can enjoy the foods you love without the mean, bad calories you hate, to instead choose the full-calorie option. If you are about my age, you have been in some way influenced by the marketing of a food industry gone awry.

It was not that long ago, when eating healthy was fairly simple—it was eating fresh, locally grown, whole foods. For most of us, our grandparents can remember eating this way. During the past few decades, we have seen a huge shift in the quality and production of what we are ingesting. We have merged the worlds of food and science and now the standard American diet consists of highly processed foods, which are packed with chemical additives, hormones, copious amounts of refined sugar, and dangerous levels of processed fats.

And it takes the simplicity out of eating. You cannot just go to a store and buy some apples. You have to find out where they are from, what they are sprayed with, if they are local, and if they are organic. I will be the first to say it: it sucks. We deserve better than to be tricked into eating stuff that might kill us. We deserve better than to be told that something is healthy, or kid-friendly, or natural, when it is actually loaded with carcinogens.

I dream of a world in which the food industry stops lying to us; in which the United States bans all the hormones, additives, and chemicals that are banned in so many other countries; and in which eating healthy is easy. But we are not there yet. We can get there through simple supply and demand. The more we educate ourselves; the more questions we ask; the more we buy the organic, fresh ingredients and leave the processed stuff rotting on the shelf; the closer we are to a future in which stores are loaded with goodness.

My client was not wrong—we should be frustrated. The food industry told her what she was eating was healthy, but she was lethargic, moody, and having extreme menopausal symptoms and bad headaches. The food industry pitches us 100-calories snack packs and fat-free yogurt, but obesity, heart disease, cancer, diabetes, depression, anxiety, and a number of other diseases are on the rise.

We need to change our approach in terms of our standard American diet or disease will continue to plague our nation. We have all heard the phrase, "you are what you eat." I am living proof that if you eat goodness, you can heal your body. It starts with educating yourself, making small changes, encouraging a healthier lifestyle, and creating a routine that becomes second nature. You have to be willing to put the work in now, ignore convenience, and take charge.

Our culture relies so heavily on convenience that it is not even considered convenience anymore—it is the status quo. So often my clients tell me that their current regime allows them about 10 minutes to make dinner and to spend any more time than that is out of the question. We have learned to ask for the biggest bang for our buck when it comes to our time.

- What gym offers the best full-body workout in the shortest amount of time?
- What service can deliver food for the cheapest amount with the least amount of assembly?
- Which therapist can offer me the most advice in the fewest number of sessions?

Our worlds are spinning faster than ever and marketing teams everywhere have found that they can sell you anything if they can make it convenient. Cue the rise of fast food, frozen dinners, pre-cut fruits and vegetables that are preserved with chemicals, and whole meals that comes from blending a packet of powder with milk in your blender. It is not all about the junk either—we are willing to pay premium pricing for someone to divide almonds into individual bags for us or to wash, peel, and chop carrots into a convenient size.

Convenience is not a bad thing when it applies to eating healthy, but the mindset of needing convenience is killing us. It convinces us that if it's not easy, we simply cannot do it. And if we cannot do it because it is not easy, then it must not be worth it. People tell me all the time, "Sure I would love to eat healthy, but I could only do it if someone grocery shopped and cooked for me."

I'm going to give you a little tough love: that is bullshit. People who have an early cancer diagnosis are lucky enough to have the opportunity to take control and change their behaviors. There are people all over the world who do not have that opportunity. People who drop dead every day because of their lifestyles or who get a cancer diagnosis that is so far progressed that there is nothing left for them to do.

Before my diagnosis, I did not think I was the picture of health, but I also did not think I was anywhere near unhealthy enough to get cancer. We think we are invincible and we think that we will change our behaviors once we are forced to. You might not be given the opportunity to make changes later, so you better make them now. And if cutting up vegetables is too inconvenient for you now, you better believe you will pay for it later.

The excuses we tell ourselves are the excuses we have been fed by brilliant marketing teams who pitch us things such as, "Who has time to make dinner these days? Buy our product and you can have fully cooked rice in 60 seconds!" You have time . . . because your health is a priority. Because you're reading this book and you care about your well-being and you have committed to stop looking for a quick fix.

Your body can only do so much for you and your health. At some point, you have to recognize that you are a team. You need each other in order to function at an optimal level. Your body and mind are continuously working, healing, and protecting your internal and external health. It cannot run on crap. You need to aid in these efforts by providing nutritious building blocks and the tools it requires to detox, heal, and thrive. In order to target cancer and other diseases, it is vital that you understand the ways in which food can both assist you as well as hurt you.

In the last chapter, I gave you my brief overview of what eating healthy means to me. Here is the wonderful thing about this lifestyle—unlike the fad diets of our past, it does not just work for some people; it works for everyone. Remember, with the 80/20 rule, it is all about balance. You can eat cake on your birthday, you can eat cheese grits when you are at the best southern restaurant in Louisiana, you can have a beer when you go to a baseball game. When you eat clean at least 80 percent of the time, it's easier for your body to get rid of the toxins that come in when you splurge. It's when your body is a buildup of constant splurging that it loses its ability to function and cleanse.

elissa goodman

Look at it this way: at least 80 percent of the time you are eating as a simple solution to not being hungry, right? So, when lunch time rolls around and your stomach is growling, you want to take action to make yourself not hungry. In that 30-minute period when you're taking a break from work and fueling your body, what is the purpose of indulging? Why eat a burger and fries (and it is not even an amazing burger and fries) when you could achieve a better, healthier end result by having a salad? You should save that burger and fries indulgence for a really amazing burger and fries and kick off your afternoon feeling energized and cleansed.

This is what I really try to explain to my clients—a cleansing, cancer-free lifestyle isn't about never indulging or stressing about every calorie that crosses your lips; it's about fueling your body with the tools and care it needs to recover from those little indulgences. Eating healthy does not mean never getting to touch dessert or eat out again, it means you make good choices today because you know you are eating out tomorrow.

Let's dive a bit deeper into my fundamental rules for eating clean.

Eat Whole Foods

In the 1980s, all I cared about was keeping my weight down. I lived off all the sugar-free and fat-free foods the grocery store could offer. SnackWell's were a personal favorite. Now, it breaks my heart a bit to even think about how much I naïvely consumed. At the time, I did not have the sense to look past the scale and notice that my energy was lacking, my mental clarity was murky, and my skin was ravaged. I never felt good after eating these foods, but I didn't connect the dots to what was causing it.

Processed foods have become such a core of the American diet. A lot of people think when I say processed foods that I'm talking about Oreos or boxed mac and cheese. Processed foods are anything that has been altered from their natural state. The yogurt you eat for breakfast, the pretzels you snack on at work, the low-calorie salad dressing you have at lunch, trail mix you have midday, the frozen pizza you pop in the oven when you are too exhausted after work to make dinner. These are all highly processed foods!

I often watch people at grocery stores. (Yes, your worst nightmare of having a nutritionist scope what you're buying is true!) I see so many carts stocked with boxes and cans, and I will assume no one buying them can pronounce most of the ingredients on those labels. It is a scary sight. People come to me all the time and tell me they do not have time to cook any other way. One of the most common situations: parents who serve frozen or packaged foods to their kids almost every night, but justify it because they give them a salad or some carrots with it.

What we are all forgetting is that there was a time in which these foods did not exist in the marketplace and people were still able to eat. The food industry has sold us convenience as a necessity and we are eating it up like fools.

We need to relearn how to eat food in its natural state. This is the post-fad diet world. Take away the gimmicks and the cool packaging and the 60-second microwave meal. We need to stop looking for calorie-free, fat-free, and sugar-free options. If it's missing fat, it's loaded with sugar. If it is missing sugar and calories, it is loaded with chemicals. We are consuming far too many foods that are empty calories—they offer zero nutrients and contribute to cancer, heart disease, diabetes, obesity, and many other life-threatening illnesses.

So, rule #1 of eating whole foods is to CUT OUT PROCESSED FOODS.

Here are the biggest offenders.

Artificial Sweeteners

Artificial sweeteners are the devil. I say this in the most genuine way possible. I have so, so much hate in my heart for artificial sweeteners because they are truly one of the worst things to happen to our country. Artificial sweeteners are the perfect example of what is wrong with our current food industry. We are so obsessed with having zero-calorie and zero-fat options that we have accepted that a powdered chemical concoction is fine to consume.

Aspartame, one of the most commonly used sweeteners is a neurotoxin, meaning it literally attacks your cells. When studied in rats, it has been shown to induce cancer in multiple regions of the body and create carcinogenic effects.

Put down the Splenda and the diet soda. It is one of the deadliest things on our market today.

Additives and Chemicals

I think sometimes this is a hard thing for people to swallow, because they cannot imagine that their government would allow the types of things that it does in our food. People look at me sometimes like I'm talking some crazy, hippy-dippy stuff when I say that our food is being poisoned. This is not a drill! There are so many products on the market that are not even really food at all!

The food we buy these days contains dozens of artificial additives and chemicals. Ever see the listed ingredient, "artificial flavors"? That "one" ingredient can account for more than 10 chemicals. Food was not supposed to be modified and preserved for months on end. What is worse is that food companies are spending millions of dollars paying scientists to come up with newer, more addictive, cheaper chemicals to add to food every day and there are no long-term studies about how safe they are. Yet, in the meantime, we have more cancer and disease than ever.

Do not allow food companies to make your diet choices for you. They are killing you and not slowly! Using wholesome, nutrient-dense ingredients is expensive for companies, which is why they are replacing them with low-quality additives and chemicals. Unlike whole foods, processed foods lack protein, healthy fats, essential carbohydrates, fiber, vitamins, and minerals. Instead of helping cancer heal, these foods fuel the problem.

Trans Fats

There have been so many fad diets, that people are confused when it comes to healthy eating and fat consumption. You absolutely, 100 percent need fat in your diet. The key is choosing the right types of fat. When you purchase processed foods, you're not gaining beneficial fats. Typically, you'll be eating large amounts of saturated and trans fats.

I had a client with cancer who was convinced that fat was still a four-letter word. He was eating a lot of low-fat and processed foods that contained trans fats. I explained to him the importance of good fats in your diet—it's a major source of energy and helps your body absorb vitamins and minerals to a higher degree. We removed the processed foods and added healthy fats to his diet. Within a week he felt more satiated, energized, and lost his desire to reach for processed foods. At his doctor's appointment a few weeks later, his inflammation, cholesterol, and blood sugar numbers had also come down a lot. He was losing weight and felt better than ever. What a simple fix!

Basically, trans fats are formed when hydrogen is added to vegetable oil. This helps it solidify and last longer. These are artificial, human-made fats, which create havoc and chaos in terms of your cellular functioning. They not only decrease immune function, but also interfere with the enzymes your body depends on to fight cancer.

Not only should you eliminate processed foods that contain trans fats, but you should also focus on incorporating healthy fats. Coconut oil, grass-fed butter, or ghee are great choices for cooking, while olive oil is highly beneficial when eaten in its raw, cold state (for example, on salads or drizzled on top of vegetables). Also, there are so many yummy healthy oils on the market today—avocado, hemp, flax, walnut, pumpkin seed, and the list goes on.

MSG

A lot of people associate monosodium glutamate (MSG) with Chinese food. It's a flavor enhancer, often known to be enhancing your takeout meal, but it is also in thousands of common household foods. It's in frozen dinners, soups, salad dressings, baby food, formulas, and more. It is known to contain carcinogenic compounds and byproducts that contribute to cancer. We have fried our taste buds with so many chemicals that they no longer can appreciate the taste of real, whole food.

We should not need dangerous additions, like MSG, to make food taste good. We need to cleanse our palettes and retrain our bodies to embrace fresh, whole foods. Even after a week or two of removing this toxic stuff, you will begin to notice how much better healthy food tastes and how unbearable the other crap tastes. Ask anyone who has ever given up sugar if she can happily eat a candy bar. I bet she will tell you it is terrible. I used to chomp on gum all day long— now if I have even half of a piece I feel sick to my stomach from all the chemicals and sugar. I cannot believe I ever chewed that all day!

MSG increases inflammation and free-radical production, which contributes to tumor growth and reduces immunity. If you're battling cancer, I'm fairly sure you want to have your immune system on your side.

These are just a few of the thousand additives that exist in our food. Synthetic flavors, colors, preservatives, high fructose corn syrup, and more have all shown to contribute to diminishing health. You have the choice: whole foods that nurture and heal your body or processed foods that attack and hurt your body?

Now that you've gotten rid of those processed foods in your life, you have room to incorporate rule #2—EAT YOUR GREENS.

One huge shift that our culture needs to make is away from the idea that vegetables are a side dish. There is no other food more nutrient dense and cancer-fighting than veggies. They should be the core of what you eat, not a side. Greens and plant-based foods are superstars in terms of preventing and treating cancer. At each meal, half of your plate should contain vegetables. At my house, we start dinner every night with a big salad.

The standard American diet has this backward, as protein and carbs tend to be the main portion while vegetables are an afterthought. Vegetables provide a huge range of antioxidants and other cancer-fighting compounds.

Phytochemicals, for instance, are plant-based chemicals that target carcinogens and reduce overall inflammation. There is an incredible natural compound called diindolylmethane (DIM) that is found in vegetables, such as mustard greens, broccoli, and cabbage. Researchers have found that this compound not only helps to prevent cancer, but also helps to treat it. Wow!

If you are someone who hates salad or the only veggie you like is glazed carrots, there is really no path to health except changing. Vegetables are non-negotiable and the most incredible food group we have! You better learn to love them. ☺

You should consume a wide variety (I always say to eat a rainbow!) as different vegetables provide different nutrients, but dark, leafy greens are a must. They are huge power players when it comes to fiber, antioxidants, carotenoids, vitamins, and minerals. If you are fighting disease of any kind or trying to prevent a diagnosis, dark, leafy greens need to be your best friend. They help target free radicals and can inhibit the growth of certain cancer types. They are incredibly effective at flushing out toxins, so your body can focus on maintaining balance and removing harmful substances from your internal systems.

If you are serious about your health, vegetables should be a part of every meal you have. I start my day with a green juice; snack on cucumbers, celery, or carrots; have a salad for lunch; a salad to start dinner; and vegetables are always at least half my dinner plate.

More than anything, vegetables are a safe bet. You can find endless research and information about how scary processed foods or dairy or gluten are online, but try finding one article about how cucumbers are bad for you or how arugula should be banned.

When you up your veggie intake, the other crap automatically gets cleansed from your diet. For starters, you don't have room but you also stop craving sugary, processed foods. It's really rather foolproof. If my publisher had asked me to write a three-word book on fighting cancer, those three words would be: EAT YOUR GREENS. In the words of Nike, just do it.

Rule #3 for eating a whole foods diet is to BUY ORGANIC.

If you just rolled your eyes at this tip, hold on one second. There are a lot of people who say buying organic is a scam and a lot of nonorganic companies are riding on the fact that there is no definitive proof that organic foods are more nutritious than nonorganic foods. So let's get to the bottom of this once and for all.

Let's take a strawberry. Strawberries are loaded with vitamin A, manganese, fiber, and iodine. There is not more vitamin A, manganese, fiber, or iodine in an organic strawberry, but here is the difference: the nonorganic strawberry has been showered in toxins and chemicals to force it to grow big and plump and preserve longer in stores. It is an extremely porous fruit so no matter how much you wash it, when you bite into a nonorganic strawberry you are biting into tons of buildup of carcinogenic toxins. We still don't know how those toxins deplete the nutritious elements of the fruits and veggies they are on, but we do know for sure that they completely counteract them.

I believe that organic provides the most nutritious option, but more important than what it provides, it is what it does NOT provide in the form of chemical pesticides. It has also been shown that plants that are given the opportunity to grow and live without being showered with fertilizers and pesticides, produce more antioxidants and vitamins, which is their natural way to improve resistance to bugs and weeds. Just like our immunity and healthy blossoms when we take care of ourselves and rid our bodies of toxins, so do theirs.

Would you put time, money, and effort into eating healthy if you were going to drink a bottle of Windex every day? There is no doubt that organic foods cost more, but they are most certainly worth their price tag. Farming has turned into a factory setting. As production increases, the quality of our food diminishes.

It is vital that you reduce your intake of toxins, especially if you have cancer. Nonorganic or conventionally grown produce are exposed to pesticides and toxins on a daily basis. You cannot cleanse your body if you are continually putting toxins back into your body.

There is a lot that needs to be done in terms of the big picture. Farmers and the products they use should be regulated and they should stop being able to expose us to countless pesticides and fertilizers that are banned everywhere else in the world. In the meantime, you can make changes as an individual. I recommend buying local and at farmer's markets as often as possible, since these crops are usually from smaller farms, which use less chemicals.

It is also true that some produce absorbs more pesticides and toxins than others, so if you can't commit to buying fully organic, here are the foods to make sure you buy organic all the time:

- strawberries
- apples
- nectarines
- peaches
- celery
- grapes
- cherries
- spinach
- tomatoes
- sweet bell peppers
- cherry tomatoes
- cucumbers

The following foods are the least affected, so if you're on a budget, these are your safest options for buying conventionally:

- avocados
- sweet corn
- pineapples
- cabbage
- sweet peas
- onions
- asparagus
- mangos
- papayas
- kiwi
- eggplant
- honeydew
- grapefruit
- cantaloupe
- cauliflower

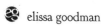 elissa goodman

In Los Angeles, we are blessed with tons of great local and organic options. When my clients ask me if it's worth the money, I always say yes, because I truly believe that, but also, it is so accessible here. We have tons of farmers markets, which offer local, organic foods at great prices. I know that it is hard to look at two apples that look seemingly the same and to choose the more expensive one. Even if money is not a problem, that still doesn't seem right.

I had a client who was resistant to the organic food movement. She felt like it was a total rip-off and she could get her body what it needed without spending like crazy. We did a bit of research and found a great farm that would deliver a fresh box of organic produce to her every week for a great price. She agreed to try it for a month and see if she felt a difference. After two weeks, she felt more energized, cleaner, and happier. I will be the first to say that maybe this was all in her head, but I think there is nothing wrong with that.

When your mind knows that you are giving your body pure goodness, this provides healing. Every time you bite into something, you should be able to say, "body, I love you, and here is this amazing pear because I respect you and want you to be able to function fully." You should not be saying, "body, I'm sorry, I want to give you goodness but I did not really want to spend the money so here is something good but it is covered in chemicals."

A study published in *Environmental Health Perspectives* found that children who eat organic fruits, vegetables, and juices can significantly lower the levels of organophosphate pesticides in their bodies. The University of Washington researchers who conducted the study concluded,

> *"Dose estimates suggest that consumption of organic fruits, vegetables, and juice can reduce levels from above to below the U.S. Environmental Protection Agency's current guidelines, thereby shifting exposure from a range of uncertain risk to a range of negligible risk. Consumption of organic produce appears*

> *to provide a relatively simple way for parents to reduce their children's exposure to OP [organophosphate] pesticides."*
>
> —CL Curl, RA Fenske, and K Elgethun
> *Environmental Health Perspectives*, March 2003

I know it is expensive but you simply cannot put a price on taking care of yourself. Cancer, diabetes, heart disease, depression, and anxiety are all way more expensive than buying organic. It never ceases to amaze me how much we allow companies and marketing to set our ideas about what a product is worth. We will pay $10 for valet, because it is standard, but not $4.50 for organic eggs because eggs are supposed to cost $3.

We are allowing companies to set the value and worth for our bodies and our health. If you want to live a cancer-free life, you have got to put your money where your mouth is. Buy the organic eggs and skip the valet—the walk from your street parking spot is good for you too!

Radically Reduce Sugar Consumption

I should have talked about sugar in the section above, where I talk about getting rid of all the bad additives and chemicals, but sugar deserves its own entire category because it is so dangerous.

Have you ever had a friend who dates a horrible guy and it is so blatantly obvious to everyone that he treats her poorly and she is not happy and it is so sad and terrible to watch? That is how I feel about sugar. I just want to shake all Americans and beg them to stop letting sugar into their lives.

In my opinion, sugar is one of the scariest things we are consuming. Sugar fuels cancer cells, which means if you are consuming it, you increase your chances of getting cancer (among other diseases). And if you have cancer, you are just encouraging it to grow. When you eat highly processed, refined sugars, it creates a dramatic spike and rapid fluctuation within your blood-glucose levels. This places stress on your body as insulin is secreted in order to try to maintain balance.

Normalizing your insulin levels is one of the most powerful physical actions you can take to lower your risk of cancer. You possess the power to starve cancer cells by eliminating sugar from your diet. There is no doubt that there are some amazing doctors out there, but it still blows my mind how few oncologists acknowledge sugar and its direct link to cancer.

There are a lot of people who think foods that are low-calorie do not have a lot of sugar in them. Sugar packs a ton of flavor for the calorie so do not think that just because your protein bar is only 100 calories that it cannot be loaded with sugar.

To reduce your risk of cancer, I would limit your intake to 25 grams of sugar per day or less. When looking at the sugar content on packages, you should aim for no more than 3 grams and not more than 5 grams per serving. This does not include eating whole fruit. I believe whole fruit is anti-cancerous. Cancer does not feed off the natural sugar in fruit, because along with the sugar are critical, natural cancer killers, such as polyphenols, resveratrol, and other antioxidants.

If I had to pinpoint the single item that is leading to the decline of our health, it is sugar. It is the most addictive, sneaky component of our current diet and most Americans consume it every single meal.

I recommend eliminating sugar from your diet, no matter what, but eating sugar if you have a cancer diagnosis is asking for trouble. Would you bring gasoline to a forest fire? Then don't bring sugar to your cancer.

Limit Animal Protein

My general rule of thumb with my family, my clients, and me is to have animal protein for one meal a day. I plan a menu for the week so everyone knows what we are having for dinner each night. If it includes an animal protein, we do not eat animal protein for lunch. The body has a hard time processing animal protein, and eating it three times a day is too much. You can have an egg for breakfast and then chicken for lunch or dinner but not for all three meals.

I have no problem with antibiotic, hormone-free, organic meat. This is another great thing to check your farmers market for! It's not chock-full of chemicals and can be a great source of protein. But you need to limit it and there are plenty of other plant-based protein sources to make sure you get your daily requirement of protein. See Appendix 1 for a list of vegan protein options.

It is also a good habit to switch it up. In my house we love chicken, turkey, bison (a great substitute for ground beef), lamb, and fish. We aim to eat red meat once a week and fish two times a week.

If you are going to eat meat, it is critical to understand how meat is currently being raised. This has a lot to do with the toxic exposure that America is facing today. Not only do you need to be concerned with how much you are consuming, you also need to know where it is coming from. Within the United States, 70 percent of all antibiotics are used on animals. This does not include all the contaminants in their food and the hormones they are injected with. This directly threatens our health and contributes to cancer. Many people ask me if there is really a difference between conventionally raised meat in comparison to organic, grass-fed, hormone-free meat. The answer is **YES**.

Cows, chickens, and pigs that are conventionally raised are fed grains that are genetically modified. This is not natural for these animals and significantly influences the end product and the people who consume it.

Contaminated meat is actually our primary source of pesticide exposure, due to the diet that the animals we eat consume. In a natural world, the diet that cattle should be consuming is grass. You might imagine that factory cattle are not eating just grass—they are loaded with corn and other plumpers, chemicals, hormones, and fillers. Yuck!

Talk to any chefs from around the world and they will tell you that the best-tasting meat is grass-fed. When you have a piece of fresh, grass-fed meat you don't need to load on marinades and flavorings to make it taste great, it just needs to be cooked. This is no coincidence! Grass-fed meat tastes the way it is intended to. It is also:

- Lower in fat.
- Higher in beta-carotene.
- Higher in B vitamins, as well as vitamin E.
- Higher in calcium, potassium, and magnesium.
- A healthier ratio of omega-3 fatty acids and omega-6 fatty acids (which is VERY important).
- Up to five times higher in conjugated linoleic acid (CLA), which is a potential cancer fighter.
- Lower in saturated fat.

You also have to be careful with fish, know where it comes from, and always buy wild-caught. Some waters are so toxic, and it is worth taking the time to research. Mercury pollution has led to increased mercury in the oceans, ultimately causing a wider variance of mercury levels in fish. Seafood has tons of health benefits, but you should make sure the fish you are eating is as nutritious and pure as possible.

As with anything, I think it is a gift to yourself to make yourself knowledgeable, but I know sometimes you can make yourself crazy trying to get all the information and the newest scoop. You cannot be perfect all of the time, make the best choice you can for yourself and move on.

There is one type of meat that you should NEVER consume and that is processed meat. Processed meats are loaded with nitrates, which

 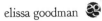

are one of the key components of our poor health and also increase our risk of certain cancers. Studies have found that just less than two ounces of processed meat daily increase your risk of cancer by a whopping 20 percent. For some cancers, this number has been reported as closer to 50–60 percent. YIKES!

We live in a Paleo world where animal protein rules what many of us consider healthy eating. It is surprisingly more common to see people who eat way too much animal protein than to see people who eat way too many carbs. We get protein from a plethora of sources—veggies, grains, lentils, beans, seeds, and nuts. It's best for our bodies to consume protein from many sources. When we overload it with one source, it cannot properly break it down and function optimally. Many people think they cannot feel full without animal protein, but I assure you a veggie-rich diet can satiate you!

One of the simplest first steps I give my clients is to limit animal protein to once a day. It will not only make you more conscious of what you are consuming throughout the day, but you will see how amazing you can feel with a diet that includes other protein sources. I'm sure you've heard this a million times before, but healthy eating is all about balance. We are not intended to live on a super protein-heavy diet and especially not all that animal protein! When I met David, he could eat a whole chicken in one sitting. If he can see the benefits of cutting back on animal protein, anyone can!

Be Smart When You Eat Out

My 21-day cleanse program is three weeks for a specific reason. When I did five-day cleanse programs in restaurants, my phone and email were always blowing up. People wanted to know what to eat before and after. They would finish the program and feel amazing and be so scared that they would eat something that would ruin the whole thing. With my 21-day program, there is a "warm-up" week, a cleanse week, and a "cool-down" week.

I love a 21-day program because it gives your body time to adapt, you create a habit, and eating that way starts to become second nature. The beauty of that is that it erases all the fear and scariness of eating out or eating something that's not spelled out for you. You start to be able to pay attention to what your body is telling you and you can order confidently.

Lots of my clients want to know one salad they can always order anywhere or the foolproof way to eat out and not mess with their diet. The truth is, it is all about getting back in touch with your body and really paying attention to what it is asking from you. Sometimes that is not a salad! Maybe you are iron deficient and you could really benefit from a lettuce-wrapped burger. Perhaps you are feeling a little wiped out and your brain could use a little salmon boost.

Eating healthy does not mean eating lettuce everywhere you go. It means listening to your body, satiating it with good, whole ingredients, and not being fooled into believing your body is asking for that basket of bread.

The 80/20 rule is so important here because it allows flexibility in your diet and life. You should enjoy food and eating and you should never feel deprived. I think splurging is really important. It takes away the power we sometimes give to food. You can have a little indulgence and it does not need to ruin your day or determine your health. The 80 percent of the time that you are eating healthy works out because it allows your body to be in tip-top shape to process the other 20 percent.

But I do have one big caveat: all splurges are not created equal. There are some items that healthy eating cannot counteract. This is something I feel like Americans are not grasping. You can eat incredibly healthy 365 days a year but if you have a diet soda vice, you are not protecting yourself against cancer. I always tell my clients, go ahead and splurge, but it better be on real, whole ingredients. A regular soda is always better than diet soda. I do not recommend that splurge because it is still sugar (bad for cancer) but it is not chemicals.

elissa goodman

If you are craving macaroni and cheese, go to the store and buy pasta, cheese, and real butter and make it. If you are craving chocolate chip cookies, go to the store and buy flour and chocolate chips and make them. If you want a candy bar, have a piece of high quality chocolate, not a candy bar.

Read the Ingredients List

If you do not know what something is on the package, do not eat it. And do not assume that if someone is selling you something— no matter how healthy it seems—that you know what is in it. Even almond milk can be loaded with cancer-causing chemicals. You can splurge, but you need to make educated choices. Every time you put something highly toxic like diet soda or other chemical-laden foods into your body, you are back to square one.

The other thing that I think is really important with splurging and eating out is to remember that giving into a craving or just the environment you're in doesn't mean you need to go totally crazy. Pizza tastes the same whether you have one slice or four. Ice cream is just as good whether you have one scoop or three. Potato chips cure that salt craving just as much with a handful as the whole bag. Don't blow your 20 percent on overeating one item. Spread it out, indulge a little here, a little there. Then it becomes less of an event and more of a lifestyle. Balance, remember?

In Appendix 2, I have included a guide about eating out and how to order at restaurants. Be sure to choose wisely to get the best food available for you at home or away.

Cut Back on Alcohol

I think this is important to talk about after we talk about splurging because a lot of people consider a cookie a splurge but not an alcoholic drink. If you're facing a cancer diagnosis, especially a tough one, I would suggest eliminating drinking any kind of alcoholic beverage. If you're trying to lose weight, cleanse, or detox, I would suggest eliminating drinking all together.

If you're just trying to be healthy and find balance, I have no problem with you having a few drinks. The overall idea here is to cut excess toxins out of your life and raise awareness about what you are consuming. If you're someone who pops open a beer or bottle of wine every day after work out of habit, it's worth stepping back and seeing if that's something you really want or need to consume.

I rarely tell my clients they cannot drink, but for those who drink regularly, I ask them to try to cut back 50 percent to start. Most of the time, what happens is they recognize the places where they consume alcohol without thinking—when they are out at dinner and have a glass of wine because everyone else does, when they stop by a friend's house and have a beer because the friend offers it, when they are at a concert and have a vodka tonic at intermission because it is available. Alcohol, like sugar, has a way of sneaking into our lives without us noticing, because a lot of times it comes with social territory. We don't even notice how often or how much we are drinking.

We can also make better choices so that when we do drink it does not send us completely off the wagon. Along with that, alcohol should be included as a splurge—part of our 20 percent. This will help us not overindulge! Sometimes the stuff we put into our bodies outside of meals can do the most damage. We need to have an honest conversation about the weight and purpose we are allowing alcohol (and other similar items) to have in our lives.

Taking a look at everything you put in your body is crucial. Sometimes there's not even a reason, you just consume because it's around or others are doing it. Committing to eating healthy is a challenge and a lot of work. It is so easy and convenient to eat junk. It's so easy to turn a blind eye to what you're eating. It is so easy to say you will begin to eat better when you make more money, or you start working different hours, or when you're less stressed.

I'm asking you to start eating healthy today. I know, it is a lot to ask. But we do not get to start saving ourselves whenever it is convenient. Look around you—people are dying from disease every single day. We see it more and more; people are literally dropping dead. We are not getting warnings or signs or red flags. We are dying.

I am so grateful that I was given the opportunity to turn my life around, but I am one of the lucky ones. I want to say I'm not trying to scare you, but I am. If you are not scared, you should be. But you are not powerless. You are in charge. So, how about that kale?

"I love myself and therefore I choose to make choices that nourish every cell of my body."

HACK 2:
An Imbalanced Gut

Did you know that the majority of the cells of your immune system (80 percent) are present in your gut? Hence, a healthy gut is critical for a healthy body.

—Dr. Ritu Goel
"21 Facts You Should Know about Your Gut," 2013

Did you know that 95 percent of the serotonin (chemical that affects happiness and well-being) and 50 percent of dopamine (chemical that affects emotions, movements, and sensations of pleasure and pain) are produced in your gut?

—Mark Sisson
"Mark's Daily Apple," 2014

Did you know that each year more than 270,000 Americans develop a cancer of the GI tract, including cancers of the esophagus, stomach, colon, and rectum? About half of these cancers result in death.

—Joseph Castro
"Live Science," 2013

I'm fairly sure every child has something that their mother says that drives them crazy. My mom used to always say to me, "Because I said so!" and I can still hear her saying it in my head all the time. For my kids, there is no doubt they would tell you that the thing I am constantly saying is, "Listen to your gut!"

elissa goodman

Well, sorry kids, but I stand by it. You have probably heard that said many times and most of you have probably shrugged it off as just something people say. In the last chapter, I said that if my publisher asked me to write a three-word book it would be "eat your greens." Well, actually I need that version of my book to be eight words and they are: "eat your greens and listen to your gut."

Think of your gut as the control center of your body. When I say, "listen to what your body is telling you," I mean it. If you think you do not know how to eat, you are wrong. Your body sends cravings based on what it needs. The problem is, those cravings are so bogged down with chemicals and other crap that they cannot get the right message to you. We are so addicted to sugar and chemicals that when our body says, "hey, I am really lacking in iron right now, could you have some spinach for lunch?" the wires are so screwy from poor diets that we instead hear, "I'm starving! Help! I need a donut!" If you are someone who finds that healthily satiating cravings are a huge problem for you, pay attention.

Taking care of your gut is the most important thing you can do for your body. Your gut health directly affects your digestive system as well as your internal and external systems. Think about the big guys—skin, brains, and heart—these are all hugely affected by your gut health. Focusing on having a healthy gut, filled with good bacteria is the first step toward more positive overall health.

When your gut is balanced, you significantly decrease your risk of disease. Here is the issue—we live in such a sterile, antibiotic-heavy culture that all the bacteria, good and bad, is wiped from our guts. We need to keep the good so that our guts can properly function. This is also why you might have noticed a huge increase in digestive issues, irritable bowel syndrome, and other stomach-related diseases. We have killed off all the good bacteria in our guts, which negatively affects so many of the systems in our bodies. We have also adopted lifestyles that help the bad bacteria to thrive. Sounds like a bit of a mess, huh?

Some of the key factors regarding bad bacteria overgrowth include:

- high levels of chronic adrenaline and stress
- a lot of negative feelings (fear, anxiety, anger, hatred, guilt, shame, etc.)
- eating too much sugar and refined carbs
- eating artificial sweeteners
- overeating animal protein
- prescription drugs, antibiotics, immunosuppressants, anti-fungals, amphetamines, etc.
- not eating enough nutrient-rich, whole foods

Additionally, there is a chemical called hydrochloric acid (HCl) that aids in the digestion of our food. The main culprits for low HCl are adrenaline, stress, negative emotions, prescription drugs, antibiotics, and overconsumption of animal protein, nuts, seeds, or legumes. Sound familiar? All of these common things are promoting the dissolution of our gut powerhouse! For my clients who are low in HCl, celery juice is incredible at restocking their systems with it. I recommend making their morning juice at least one-third celery juice to help with digestion and rebuilding their HCl.

Okay, so what is the big deal with gut health? Approximately 70 percent of our immune system is found within our guts. So when our gut fails, so does our immunity and when our immunity fails, so does our health and our ability to combat cancer. Poor gut health means your defenses are down and your body cannot protect you. This leads to inflammation and a weakened state, which leaves you more susceptible to cancer.

If you are being treated for cancer, positive gut health is crucial. You must strengthen your immune system or your body will break down and you will be incredibly prone to other viruses and diseases. When I lost my husband, Marc, it was not to cancer, it was to pneumonia because the chemotherapy had thoroughly depleted his immune system. I see this happen all the time!

Did you see the film *Dallas Buyers Club?* Based on a true story, Matthew McConaughey's character has AIDS and starts taking a new popular drug at the time that claims it can cure it. What happens is this pill wipes out ALL the bacteria, so, yes—it takes the bad stuff with it, but it also takes the good stuff. He recognizes that people all around him who are on this medication are dying because their bodies are so depleted from this pill that they cannot fight off simple viruses. It is not adding years or vitality to their lives.

The drug company can get away with this because these people are not dying from AIDS anymore, so technically the pill has done its job. Scary. McConaughey's character starts fueling his body with vitamins, supplements, and a healthy diet. He ends up living another seven years when originally he was given only a few weeks to live.

I might have been the only person in that theatre in Los Angeles thinking about how pertinent this story was to the cancer fight, but it is an amazing example of how what you eat, how you treat your body, and giving care to your gut health and immunity can change a death sentence to living life.

I feel so passionately about gut health and it is important to me that if you are reading this book that you understand what a huge influence your gut has on your body and health. This is not the chapter to skim!

Here are some ways to get your gut in check and your health on track.

Reduce Toxic Trigger Foods

I have echoed this sentiment a lot, but it is important for you to understand how foods can either help or hurt you. With your gut, there are foods you can eat to improve gut health. No surprise here—the gut demands whole, nutrient-dense foods, but it also thrives on fermented foods, which I will further talk about later in this chapter.

But more important than that is the massive negative effect a bad diet has on the gut. For most of us, the way we eat has destroyed our guts. On top of that, antibiotics, birth control, acne medication, alcohol, stress, and other toxins ruin our gut health. These factors cause inflammation in your gut, impeding its ability to function and serve as the powerful control for the rest of your body. Removing these factors can significantly improve your overall health.

When you eat refined grains, sugar, and processed foods, they are feeding the bad bacteria, allowing them to rapidly multiply. In our antibiotic culture, we are wiping the good bacteria from our systems so we are left with an overgrowth of the bad and none of the good. Our bodies not only need the good bacteria, but they also need the bad bacteria to be kept in check.

Currently, millions of people are suffering from a huge imbalance of microorganisms and yeast overgrowth. As a society, we eat far too much sugar and starches. Since bad bacteria feed on sugar, you should not eat ANY refined sugars and especially high fructose corn syrup.

Another big factor is how much omega-6 fatty acids we tend to consume. These are the bad fatty acids and they increase inflammation and digestive complications. Eliminating processed foods from your diet will help with this, but the best thing you can do is to cut out all processed vegetable oils (soy, corn, canola, safflower) and replace them with coconut oil, raw olive oil, nut oils, ghee, and butter from grass-fed cattle.

In a major study in the *Journal of the American Medical Association*, hidden gluten sensitivity was shown to increase risk of death by 35 to 75 percent, mostly by causing heart disease and cancer. By just this mechanism alone, more than 20 million Americans are at risk for heart attack, obesity, cancer, and death. Dairy and gluten are the most common triggers of food allergies that are linked to insulin resistance. Cutting them out of the diet allows the inflamed gut and an inflamed body to heal.

Add Fermented Probiotic Foods

Probiotic foods are excellent for maintaining a healthy gut. The beneficial bacteria in probiotic foods are some of the same bacteria that populate a healthy gut, so when you eat these foods, it's an infusion of healthy flora right where they need to be.

I love a probiotic supplement, which I talk a bit more about later in this chapter, but I am always a huge advocate for getting as much as possible from your foods. Supplements are incredible and I use a ton of them, but they should be treated exactly as their name implies, as supplements, not as stand ins. I always encourage my clients to add foods that naturally supply what a supplement would and then add in a supplement to boost that effort.

You never know the life a supplement lives before it reaches you! If it gets stuck on a hot truck for weeks at a time with no refrigeration, the end result could be an expensive placebo. So, as a rule of thumb, reach for foods first, supplements second. Better to be overloaded with goodness than relying on a pill.

There's no risk of taking a placebo with probiotic foods, especially if you make them yourself, because if they had no bacteria, they wouldn't ferment in the first place. You can be sure that the bacteria are actually there, because you watched them transform ordinary cabbage into delicious sauerkraut.

There are a few fermented, probiotic-rich foods, which I highly encourage adding to your regular diet:

- **Bragg Organic Apple Cider Vinegar**—For centuries in the natural health community, this vinegar has been used as an ancient folk remedy, claimed to help with all sorts of health issues and especially digestion. It is important to use raw, unpasteurized apple cider vinegar, because it contains strands of "mother," which means it's unprocessed, living vinegar.

- **Yogurt**—I'm not a big fan of dairy so I don't encourage eating a lot of yogurt, but if you feel like you want it, I only recommend organic, all-natural, unsweetened, Greek or goat's milk yogurt with live and active cultures. My all-time favorite is nondairy coconut yogurt kefir, which I make with fresh coconut meat.

- **Organic Coconut Water Kefir**—This fermented coconut water contains high concentrations of beneficial bacteria that aid in digestion.

- **Organic Tempeh**—Tempeh is an amazing probiotic-rich meat supplement. You must make sure the tempeh you are choosing is non-GMO, but since it's fermented, I prefer it to tofu. I add it to salads, stir-fry recipes, wraps, and more for a protein, probiotic, and vitamin B12 boost.

- **Kimchi**—An Asian staple, kimchi is a delightful sour and spicy fermented cabbage. As long as your body can handle spicy foods, kimchi is an incredible probiotic addition to your diet.

- **Unpasteurized Organic Miso**—A "living food" containing natural digestive enzymes, beneficial bacteria, and other microorganisms that aid in the digestion of all foods and have been shown to ward off and destroy harmful microorganisms, thereby creating a healthy digestive system.

- **Sauerkraut**—A German word, sauerkraut translates to "sour cabbage." Not only does this fermented cabbage fuel healthy gut bacteria but it contains choline, a chemical needed for the proper transmission of nerve impulses in the brain and throughout the central nervous system.

There was a study done about Polish women and breast cancer rates. The researchers compared women who lived in Poland with women who had emigrated from Poland to the United States. The women who lived in Poland ate three times as much raw sauerkraut as the other women and the study found that their cancer rates were actually one-third of the other women. Sauerkraut contains high concentrations of glucosinolates, which have been shown to create anti-cancer effects. See? The power of food!

Add Prebiotics Foods

Prebiotic foods are like fuel for good bacteria. They are a type of nondigestible fiber compound that pass through the upper part of the GI tract and remain undigested since the human body cannot fully break them down. Once they pass through the small intestine, they reach the colon, where they're fermented by the gut microflora. They have certain fibrous carbohydrates that nourish the good bacteria to help them grow. This process helps build a healthy microbiome, which is our defense system against toxins we encounter from animal products, the environment, poor quality tap water, and common yeast and viruses or other types of fungi.

Nature gave us quite the gift when it comes to prebiotic foods because there are many that have just the right "ingredients" to improve gut function without us having to do anything else but eat them! You can pair them with other probiotic foods for an even better result, or just include several of them throughout the day, separately from your probiotic-rich foods. Prebiotics work together with probiotics to preserve and maintain the balance and diversity of intestinal bacteria and to increase the presence of good bacteria. You just can't get enough!

Here are some of my favorite prebiotic foods: apples, asparagus, bananas, onions, garlic, cabbage, beans, legumes, bran, artichokes, leeks, and root veggies (sweet potatoes, squash, wild yams, jicama, beets, carrots, turnips, and parsnips).

Prebiotic foods are a source of soluble fiber. This takes us to the importance of fiber in your diet for a healthy gut. Make sure you get enough fiber daily—25 grams for women and 38 grams for men. Fiber plays a major role in digestive health. Fiber is the fuel the colon cells use to keep them healthy. Fiber also helps to keep the digestive tract flowing, removing toxins, extra hormones, and keeping your bowel movements regular. My favorite sources are beans; legumes; raspberries; collard, turnip, and beet greens; quinoa; millet; broccoli; spinach; cinnamon; soaked chia seeds; and ground flaxseeds. (I talk more about the importance of fiber in the "parasite" chapter.)

Remember, your body tells you when it's running properly. You should expect it to run like a well-oiled machine and it wants to! If something feels funky or clogged, there's an issue.

Add Bone Broth

Broth is a traditional food that your grandmother likely made often (and if not, your great-grandmother definitely did). Many societies around the world still consume broth regularly, as it is an inexpensive and highly nutrient dense food.

The secret behind the power of bone broth is collagen, the main supportive proteins that give bone, cartilage, and tendons their strength. Once cooked it becomes "gelatin." Supplementing with collagen or gelatin is important because it can help boost your gastric juices and aid in repairing the integrity of your intestinal walls.

Add Supplements

You could drive yourself a bit crazy trying to take all the supplements that I could recommend. There are so many incredible products nowadays that I have a hard time not wanting to try everything! When I find a great product, you better believe I'm spreading the word. But that can be a bit much and supplements (just as their title suggests) are there to add to and complement a healthy, nutrient-dense diet.

Here's the thing with supplements. Personally, I love and utilize them often. Some women have a closet full of shoes. I have a closet full of supplements! When my kids or my fiancé come home with a cold, I load them up on tons of supplements and herbs. But that's because I have them and I like to use them. You don't need to buy or use every supplement I mention in this book. Find the ones that speak to you, focus on the issues you feel need your attention and start there. You can always add more or try something different.

Every single one of you is different and a supplement that was life changing for me might not work as well for you. I am offering a lot of options not to overwhelm or discourage you, but to give you alternatives if you don't get the results you want from some of them. So use these lists and mark down what speaks to you, but also feel free to take them with a grain of Himalayan Pink salt. ☺

Take a Probiotic

When my clients tell me to keep their list of supplements simple, this is at the top of the list. Taking a daily probiotic ensures you have healthy levels of good bacteria in your gut, helping it properly function. Your lifestyle, toxins, chemicals, stress, chlorinated water, and polluted air can all affect your gut bacteria without you even noticing. Having your gut functioning at top model not only improves digestion and your overall health, it also increases the absorption of nutrients.

Please remember that, as with all supplements and vitamins, not all products are created and manufactured equally. Do your research and make sure you are buying from a reputable source and choosing options that are dairy-free and contain live bacteria. This will help break down your food, boost your gut, and improve overall immunity.

There are a few things to look for when buying a probiotic supplement, you want one with the different strains of probiotic bacteria, because they have slightly different functions and are concentrated in various places along the digestive tract. They tend to be more effective overall than products containing an extremely high concentration of just one or two strains. This is because many strains work synergistically to influence our health. The whole literally is greater than the sum of its parts.

In my opinion, the best probiotic supplements will include at least these three most important strains:

- **L. acidophilus**—This is the most important strain of the Lactobacillus species and it readily colonizes on the walls of the small intestine. It supports nutrient absorption and helps with the digestion of dairy foods.

- **B. longum**—Like L. acidophilus, Bifidobacterium longum is one of the most common bacteria found in the digestive tracts of adults, and it helps maintain the integrity of the gut wall. It is particularly active as a scavenger of toxins.

- **B. bifidum**—This strain, found in both the small and large intestine, is critical for the healthy digestion of dairy products. This is especially important as you grow older and your natural ability to digest dairy declines. B. bifidum also is important for its ability to break down complex carbohydrates, fat, and protein into small components that the body can use more efficiently.

I also recommend switching up your probiotic supplement every few months to give your body exposure to a wide range of strains. Check out the probiotics I recommend in Appendix 3.

Take a Digestive Enzyme

In order to properly process and digest your food, you require a healthy supply of digestive enzymes. These enzymes help break down larger molecules, so that they become more easily digestible. Your digestive enzymes are highly specialized; there are certain ones to break down fats, another to break down proteins, others to break down carbohydrates, and others to break down cellulose into simple sugars.

The problem is that it is incredibly common for your storage of enzymes to become depleted. Inflammation, stress, food sensitivity, and other problems can affect your digestive enzyme supply. It's really important for the digestive process to work as our body can only absorb nutrients if the nutritious food we eat is properly digested. Digestive enzymes take a meal with lots of properties (amino acids, fatty acids, sugars, carbohydrates, vitamins, minerals, and other elements) and break it down so the body can properly absorb, store, and utilize these elements.

Take broccoli, for instance. Once you eat it, it needs to be broken down so that the amino acids, vitamins, and minerals it provides can be absorbed. The gut is a good reminder that eating healthy is just the first step. You need to be sure that your body can properly absorb and use these nutrients.

Raw foods contain live enzymes, which help break down the food before it hits the digestive system. Yet, when you consume a lot of processed foods and not a lot of raw, organic foods, you place immense stress on your body and health. Your body no longer possesses the ability to break down your food. So, if you have a diet that includes processed foods, when you *do* eat healthy foods, your body might not be able to even use the nutrients it's providing.

One great tip is to really chew your food well. Don't just gulp or swallow what you put in your mouth. It needs to be given a good start by taking time to chew it into a smaller, ready-to-digest pulp. The enzymes in your saliva are a great way to start this process. This will signal increased enzyme production and is a great habit to get into.

While chewing boosts digestion, the more surefire way to benefit increased enzymes is to take digestive enzyme supplements. This improves and speeds up digestive reactions, aiding in overall gut health.

Take a L-Glutamine Supplement

Typically, I would never recommend so many supplements for one focus, but gut health is so important and there are so many supplements that can benefit the gut without posing harm to any other part of your body. L-glutamine is an amino acid, which can positively impact intestinal health. Your intestinal cells love this stuff, as it helps build and repair gut lining and restore your gut's integrity. If you have gut inflammation currently, I highly recommend adding this supplement to your routine (3–5 grams daily).

The gut is naturally permeable to small molecules in order to absorb these vital nutrients. In fact, regulating intestinal permeability is one of the basic functions of the cells that line the intestinal wall. In sensitive people, gluten can cause the gut cells to release zonulin, a protein that can break apart tight junctions in the intestinal lining. Other factors—such as infections, toxins, stress, and age—can also cause these tight junctions to break apart.

Once these tight junctions get broken apart, you have a leaky gut. When your gut is leaky, things like toxins, microbes, undigested food particles, and more can escape from your intestines and travel throughout your body via your bloodstream. Your immune system marks these "foreign invaders" as pathogens and attacks them.

There are a few brands of L-Glutamine that I love, and I have those listed in Appendix 3.

Take Herbs to Support Your Gut

If you are suffering from on-going gut issues, I love using herbs for their antimicrobial effect for the gut as they reduce yeast, bacteria, and parasites. These can be used in order to reduce pathogenic bacteria and restore balance in the gut. I have picked my top four favorites that are beneficial and supportive for most gut issues. As I mentioned before, you do not need to take all of these; rather if you are suffering from gut issues, find one or two that works for you!

- **Oregano Oil**—It is one of the most powerful natural antifungals, so oregano oil is an excellent choice of antifungal to start your Candida treatment. Oregano oil is not only an antifungal, but also has antiviral, antibacterial, and anti-inflammatory properties. One study has even shown it to have cancer-preventative properties too.

- **Grapefruit Seed Extract**—The 1990 study of grapefruit seed extract (published in the *Journal of Orthomolecular Medicine*) found GSE to be "highly effective against different yeasts and molds." Its antifungal properties help it to combat Candida infestations by killing the yeast cells in your intestines.

  "The great thing about taking grapefruit seed extract for digestive complaints is that it leaves the beneficial bacteria in your system intact. Compare that to other antimicrobial treatments that can leave your intestine empty of these helpful organisms."

  —The Candida Diet website

- **Garlic Extract**—Garlic is a natural immune booster and antibiotic. By taking garlic extract, you consume more than 100 active compounds. Garlic is incredible and associated with a reduced risk of various cancers, including colon, stomach, pancreas, breast, and esophagus.

- **Aloe Vera**—Due to its high enzymatic content; its antibacterial, antifungal, and antiviral properties; and the fact that it is a powerful anti-inflammatory, aloe vera is great for anyone suffering from digestive complaints.

My favorite brands of these supplements are listed in Appendix 3.

I also want to remind you how important it is to eat peacefully and mindfully. Our mental and emotional attitude while we feed our bodies directly helps with digestion. If you eat or drink something and you focus on the good in it, you will truly feel a difference. Showing gratitude toward the things you consume might sound silly, but it alerts your body that you are making positive choices with intention. When you drink a green juice and think, "I love myself and I'm loading my body with these amazing greens to kickstart a positive and healthy day," your body feels that energy and matches its objective. If you just gulp something down as if it's a chore, your body will match that as well. Many of my clients have laughed at me for this and every one of those people have come back to me and said they did notice a difference when they changed their mindset. Positivity, awareness, and gratitude go a long way!

Another tip I give people when it comes to digestion is to drink a lot of water during the day, but not during a meal. I have found that drinking water during my meals dilutes the digestive enzymes and nutrients. I encourage my clients to drink water before and after the meal but focus on the food during. You might notice that your body has a better ability to digest and break down the food and you feel better once you're done eating.

Our bodies are all so unique that often times when I meet with clients and we try to pinpoint a problem area, it takes a time or two to really nail it. There are so many elements at play that there's never one guaranteed reason why one might be feeling crappy or gaining weight or not sleeping. But there's one thing we can all do to better our health and that's to take care of our guts. We can only benefit by feeding our bodies good bacteria and helping everything run smoothly. If you are serious about taking control of your health, you must start in your gut.

"I trust my body to tell me what it needs and I honor what it tells me."

HACK 3:
Water

Did you know that 41 percent of American teenagers display visible signs of excessive fluoride exposure?

—US Centers for Disease Control and Prevention, May 2015

Did you know that distilled water increases the amount of toxic contaminants in your water?

—Dr. Joseph Mercola, Mercola.com, December 2013

Did you know that unfiltered tap water can actually increase your risk of cancer based on the toxins and chemicals you're exposed to?

—*The Huffington Post*, July 2012

As someone who has committed my life to nutrition and holistic living, I know how easily it is to be scared by something you once thought of as healthy. My biggest critics are the people who say, "Oh, come on, everything gives you cancer nowadays!" To an extent, I understand that. Our lives often feel doomed.

Here we are, a developed country and yet our government is allowing our children to eat carcinogenic-laced fruit snacks, and we are encouraged to buy skin scream that gives us skin cancer. Poisons are in our snacks, in our clothes, in our food containers, in our medicine, and in the air. Every day there's a new study released that sheds light on another everyday item that might cause cancer. Kind of makes you want to give in and buy a pack of cigarettes and a big bag of Cheetos, doesn't it?

elissa goodman

I get it. How can we keep up? And how can we ever know if these new studies present truth or if it's just another marketing scam? In a lot of ways, I think we are lucky. We are at the forefront of a changing world. What we were doing wasn't working. We are fatter, sadder, and dying faster. Our state of being has inspired a change. That's step one.

Step two is making that change the norm. That won't be today and it won't be tomorrow. There will be lots of people for years to come who will continue believing that gluten-free is a scam and aspartame won't kill you. But a little time will pass, and we will learn big lessons along the way. We will educate ourselves and we will educate our children. We will make better choices and see better results. We will become healthier, happier, and we will live long lives. And the tide will turn and this will be the norm.

Until then, the naysayers will continue. But that is okay. I have seen miracles happen from people who have holistically addressed their physical, mental, and emotional health. I am here today because I did it myself. So, if you're skeptical, all I can tell you is that doing all the stuff I recommend cannot hurt you. I'm not asking you to take any wild pills or do anything extreme. But if you're skeptical, as a caveat: this chapter might bug you.

The thing I always tell my clients is that none of this journey is about me. It's about them and no matter what I do or say, *they* need to want to change and *they* need to believe they can. If you come into my office harping about how there's nothing wrong with eating dairy at every meal and you don't care what my dumb research shows, guess what—change is not going to come.

I had a new client once who came in stubborn as could be. His sessions with me were a gift from his daughter who was concerned about his health and I could tell he did not want to be there. We went through the red flags in his diet and he looked up at me and said, "oh, and let me guess, water causes cancer too?" Well, he wasn't exactly the best audience for this answer, but I could not lie: yes, water is a concern too. I never saw him again.

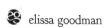 elissa goodman

The only time I ever lose clients is when they are not ready to hear what I'm telling them, and that is totally okay. I cannot help someone who does not truly want to be helped. It's easy to say something is crazy when you don't want to do it. I get that and I've done it myself. It's a guard we put up that simply says, "I am not ready to hear that."

I totally get that some of us aren't ready to hear that water is an issue! Water feels like the simplest form of health. We all know we need it, most of know we need a lot of it, and considering it's calorie-free, gluten-free, carb-free, nonfat, sugar-free, paleo, vegan, etc., it feels fairly harmless.

I really hate to be the bearer of bad news and the last thing I want to do is instill fear inside of you, but water is worrisome.

Most of us grew up drinking right from the tap. Now, most homes have some sort of filter or fridge system. I want to be extremely clear: we are so, so lucky to have access to water. Although the water we have in the United States is considered clean, our tap water is often contaminated. If you're focusing on a whole food, nutrient-rich diet, it's easy to overlook the water that's flowing out of your tap. Unfortunately, there's a wide range of contaminants and pollutants that directly threaten your health.

Here are the heavy hitters:

Arsenic

Within the United States, the level of arsenic in the water is fairly high. As I'm sure you're aware, this element is toxic to humans. It is a powerful carcinogenic, that is no stranger to cancer development. Shockingly, it's estimated that 56 million Americans are currently drinking water that contains unsafe arsenic levels. Yikes!

In terms of cancer, arsenic is a carcinogen, plain and simple. This means, that it either causes cancer or helps cancer develop and grow. It's believed that this might be due to the ways in which

 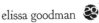

carcinogenic substances damage one's genome, while disrupting cellular metabolic processes.

Although most areas will claim that arsenic levels are low, long-term exposure can cause cancer. Most commonly, these cancers will develop in the lungs, bladder, kidneys, and skin. Since arsenic has no taste, odor, or color, it often goes unnoticed.

Aluminum

Although the levels are said to be low, there is no doubt that many people are consuming aluminum each and every day. Aluminum tends to be associated with Alzheimer's disease, however it's also known to have negative effects on various other organs and systems.

You might have heard of the potential link between antiperspirants and breast cancer. This belief is due to the concentration of aluminum. Basically, aluminum compounds "plug" your sweat ducts. Dangerous substances and compounds are then trapped in the body. Although there is still some debate about this matter, there's no doubt that aluminum is damaging to the human body. Back to my original argument—you can either take the huge risk that it will give you cancer if you are exposed to it or you can remove the risk by removing the substance and the worst-case scenario is you are cancer-free and too cautious.

Fluoride

Your dentist is not going to like me for this, and the jury is still out, but more and more is being uncovered about the dangers of fluoride. Some cities are now offered a choice about whether or not fluoride is added to their water. I personally feel strongly that this will be one of those things we deemed safe (like cigarettes) and we will look back and be scared about how wrong we were.

There's a really incredible doctor whom I admire that is recognized as the worldwide leader regarding this topic. He is incredibly

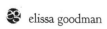

passionate about eliminating fluoride from public drinking water and if anyone knows, he does. Here are his main arguments:

- Fluoride is NOT a nutrient and it does not benefit any internal processes.
- Once it is added to the water system, there's no way of controlling doses. Nothing is being done to control factors such as age, health, or weight in regard to consumption.
- Fluoride is known to be toxic, even at low levels.
- Fluoride accumulates in bones, which could potentially lead to frail and brittle bones.
- Although it's supposed to treat dental decay, the FDA has not approved fluoride. It is currently classified as an **unapproved drug.**
- Fluoride is believed to affect brain health, which is why there's growing concerns for degenerative conditions like Parkinson's and Alzheimer's, regarding fluoride consumption.

Okay, so you're probably a bit grossed out and scared about the stuff in your water. These are the main offenders, but every city has different water content Right now you're probably thinking about all the water you drink, but you also need to keep in mind that this is the same water we shower and bathe in, the same water we wash our dishes in, and the same water we wash our clothes in.

So here comes the part where I tell you how to fix it, right? I'm going to be honest with you, this is the area in which I feel the least secure in offering you a solution. There are a lot of people who tell me they can't afford to eat organic or buy vitamins. I have found that there is always a way to make that work on any budget. The problem with water is that there aren't really any accessible options that make a huge difference. Yes, at a minimum, you should use some sort of over-the-counter water filtration system, like a Brita. No, that won't get everything. Ideally, you could install a filtration system on all the water in your house but that's an expensive project.

I talk a lot to my clients about doing the best they can. One of the worst things we can do is criticize or shame ourselves for our choices. We all make mistakes, we all have limits and slip ups and moments of weakness. It's when we think if we can't get 100 percent, we might as well fail the test. How about shooting for a B? Something is always better than nothing.

So, when it comes to water, I'm going to be real with you. The best option isn't that accessible but the worst option can be prevented. Get a filter on your shower and a filter for the water you drink. If possible, install a filter on your faucets for your dishes. If you can afford it, get the whole house filter. If you can't, don't stress.

I do a cleanse program for LA people and one of the drinks on the cleanse is my detox tonic. A wonderful little store in LA asked me to use this water it carries called intention water in my tonic. The specific water was called "love water" and was blessed with feelings of love. It was really an incredible experiment. The first few weeks of my cleanse, I didn't use the love water and not one customer said anything about the detox tonic. When I started using the love water, emails came flooding in. My assistant and I couldn't believe it! Almost everyone commented on how much they loved the detox tonic and how good it made them feel. A coincidence? I think not!

There's a lot of intention in everything we do and consume. If you drink something and you focus on the good of it, you will feel a difference. In my office, I have a wonderful brand of water called Mountain Valley Mineral Water. I can truly feel it within my body when I drink it. I love this water and it loves me right back. If all you have is a Brita, drink that water like it's Mountain Valley water. Feel it nourishing your insides, hydrating your organs and purifying your body. Maybe that feels like a cop-out but sometimes that's the best we can do.

I do have a few water rules, so whatever your filter situation, grab a glass and pay attention:

Bottled Water Is Not What It Seems

For many years, people have turned their concern with tap water toward a bottled-water drinking revolution. You can now buy dozens of different brands of bottled water, but for the most part, **it's a scam.**

Sources estimate that 25–40 percent of bottled water is just tap water. This is something I personally really hate because when you're out to lunch or on a plane or at a concert, bottled water feels like the healthy option, right? You've chosen to avoid the soda and the alcohol and then the bottled water option is crappy too! It sucks.

Worse than that, it's bottled in plastic that contains the lethal BPA chemical. BPA is a known hormone disruptor found in tons of plastic products. BPA has been linked to infertility, diabetes, obesity, and other awful diseases. We need to be taking this more seriously. Everyone still drinks bottled water like crazy! Manufacturers will now mark items if they are "BPA free" but that doesn't mean they are okay for you; it just means there's some other similar chemical with a different name in there.

On top of all that, bottled water is terrible for the environment. I use reusable steel or glass bottles. They are better for the environment and better for your health! Make a habit to always have one with you and in your bag. This is one of those simple steps, that once you create the habit, you'll never find yourself reaching for a toxic bottle of water again.

Drink Half Your Bodyweight in Ounces Each Day

If you are thirsty, you are already immensely dehydrated. We are so used to ignoring the symptoms of dehydration, we don't even realize we are suffering from it. So many people who come to me with headaches or fatigue issues are actually just dehydrated. Water—what a simple fix. Chronic dehydration can lead to digestive complications, hindered waste elimination, urinary tract infections, chronic fatigue syndrome, weight gain, and premature aging.

The most common recommendation is to drink six eight-ounce glasses a day but we are all different. My recommendation is to drink AT LEAST half your bodyweight in ounces daily. So if you are 150 pounds, you need to drink, at minimum, 75 ounces of water every day. As always, you need to be paying attention to your body. For days that you are active or it's really hot, you need to drink more.

Let Your Urine Be Your Guide

Our urine is the eyes to our water soul. Our kidneys are incredible; they filter gallons upon gallons of water. They work really hard to filter out excess water and waste, protecting you against illness and toxic buildup. On average, your urine is 95 percent water and 5 percent substances that your body wants to eliminate. Normal urine will be clear in color with a slight straw-yellow tinge.

There are a lot of factors that can affect your urine, however. Time of day, diet, medications, and water intake will change the way your urine looks. Maybe it's a little TMI, but I love looking at my urine and trying to see what my body is telling me. If you're gross and curious like me, here's a little chart to help you decipher:

Color	What Does It Mean?
Transparent	You're drinking enough water. If your urine continuously has no color, you might even want to cut back on water consumption.
Pale Straw Color— Transparent Yellow	You are healthy and normal and this indicates proper hydration. No further action is required at this point.

Dark Yellow— Light Orange	Although still normal, you should drink some water. Different hues of yellow will indicate different levels of hydration. Once your urine becomes dark yellow, this is an early sign of dehydration. If you do consume more water and an orange hue persists, contact your doctor.
Honey Color	Once your urine reaches an amber color, you should immediately drink water. This indicates that you're most certainly dehydrated, which can often result from intense heat or exercise.
Brownish Color	This could either be based on SEVERE dehydration or even liver disease. If this coloration persists after hydration, please see your doctor and have your urine sample examined immediately.
Pink or Red	Although some foods might influence your urine color (dark berries and beets for example), this could be serious. You might have blood in your urine, which could be from a urinary tract infection, kidney complications, prostate issues, or something else. You need to contact your doctor at this point. It's always better to be safe, taking the necessary steps to ensure positive health.

Now tell me you aren't going to look at your pee tonight! ☺

Not All Liquids Are Hydrating

I am always blown away by how many people still don't understand that drinks like soda and energy drinks aren't hydrating. In fact, they dehydrate you! These drinks provide a short burst of energy by raising your glucose levels but eventually you will crash. Sports drinks and vitamin waters are loaded with artificial flavors, colorants, high fructose corn syrup, and other chemicals. We are fooled into thinking that sports drinks are necessary for high-intensity workouts but the truth is they are just Kool-Aid-type drinks with salt added.

A friend of mine often tells the story of how she was working at an outdoor exercise conference on a really hot weekend in LA. One of her colleagues was super busy and running around and sweating a ton. She saw him multiple times down an entire water bottle in one gulp. A little while later she saw him with a group of people and he suddenly went into shock and couldn't even speak. Everyone was screaming to get him water, as he was clearly overheated.

She knew that he had been drinking a ton of water already and that's not what he needed. Her nursing degree kicked in; she grabbed some pretzels and tried to feed them to him. As you might imagine, he did not want to eat pretzels and she said he almost punched her in the face! But she forced them down and he immediately recovered. When it's super-hot out, we do need a ton of water but we also need salt to help us retain it.

The best thing you can do during a high-intensity workout is add a touch of natural, unprocessed Himalayan salt to your water. This will provide you with the minerals to enhance optimal functioning. I also love coconut water as a replacement for energy drinks, it's a million times more nourishing without the other crap.

While the jury is still out on carbonated water, I personally don't like it. I feel like it disrupts your body's balance. Plus, often times sparkling water is "enhanced" with added chemicals, sweeteners, sodium, etc. In my opinion, carbonated water is not a replacement for water, so if you have a little carbonated addiction, don't feel like that counts against your daily water count.

There are only a few water filters and filtering methods that I would recommend. You can use a pitcher, a faucet-mount, a faucet-integration, a counter-top filter, an under-sink filter, or a whole-house water filter.

Filtering methods include: carbon-activated carbon filters, deionization/ion exchange filters, and reverse osmosis filters. Let's discuss each method.

Carbon-Activated Carbon Filters

Activated carbon binds with many contaminants and removes them from water. It can remove asbestos, chlorine, lead, mercury, and volatile organic compounds (VOCs). But, carbon filters cannot remove arsenic, fluoride, nitrate, or percholate. Their effectiveness varies widely by manufacturer—some might only remove chlorine.

Deionization/Ion Exchange Filters

An ion exchange filter can remove heavy metals, minerals, and charged ions. It cannot remove chlorine byproducts, microorganisms, or VOCs.

Reverse Osmosis Filters

Reverse osmosis filters use a semi-permeable membrane that can trap any molecule bigger than water. They are more effective than carbon filters since they are able to remove fluoride. A reverse osmosis filter is my personal recommendation for the kind of water filter that is best.

Water is complicated because it's not something like gluten that you can just cut out completely. Not only must we drink water, but we bathe in it, swim in it, clean with it. I hate having things in which I can't lead my clients to a specific solution. It feels like a weird,

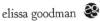

elissa goodman

fuzzy zone in which nothing is clear and therefore it's hard to make any progress at all. But in a way, water represents a microcosm of my lifestyle. It's not black and white and it's not always easy. What it always comes down to is trusting your gut and making the best decision you can make in that moment. If something doesn't feel right, make a different choice. You cannot be perfect all the time. Inevitably you will be at your kid's soccer game, dehydrated and forced to buy a bottle of water. It's okay. Buy the bottle, get hydrated, make a mental note to grab a glass bottle from your fridge next time and move on. This isn't about shaming you for the choices you make or the water pitcher you have; it's about learning and progress. You're doing great.

> *"With every glass of water I drink, I feel refreshed, replenished, healthy, and vibrant."*

HACK 4:
Parasites

*Did you know that parasites are the most common
form of life on Earth?*

—US Centers for Disease Control and Prevention, August 2012

*Did you know that there are more than 80,000 types of
protozoa (single-celled organisms), which are the
deadliest human parasites?*

—Healthline, May 2013

*Did you know that more than 50 million American children
are currently living with worm parasites, however only a small
fraction will be detected and reported?*

—Integrative Health, May 2012

We all have one story we would rather never talk about again. The story we want to disappear from our memories so that we never feel compelled to share it or remember it ourselves. Maybe it makes your skin curl or stomach twirl or head feel woozy. For me, the story I am about to share does all of the above. It is hands down the grossest thing that has ever happened to me. It's taken all the strength I have to share it with you, because instead of publishing it in my book, I'd like to find someone who can remove the image from my brain.

I had not yet been diagnosed with cancer, but I had just moved from New York to Los Angeles. I was having some digestive issues. Of course, at that time I was not thinking that the food I was eating could play into my digestive issues, but I digress.

elissa goodman

I decided to go get some colonics and see if that would help with my digestion. After my second colonic, I was in the shower and I felt something come out of my butt. Oh, cue the skin curling and stomach twirling. I cannot ever explain to you how freaky a feeling it was to feel this and then look back and pull out a parasite that was at least a foot long. As you might imagine, I totally panicked—I couldn't even tell if this thing was living or dead. There is no feeling quite like pulling something potentially living out of your body! I am not the type of girl who can handle this kind of thing happening. I was screaming bloody murder.

Thankfully, Marc was home and was able to remain calm enough to put the parasite into a plastic bag so we could take it to the hospital and figure out what the heck it was. I had never felt so gross in a shower before.

The doctor told us that it was a fairly common parasite but that my colonic sessions had induced it to come out my body. I have to admit, there's a part of me that wishes it had just stayed in there. Though I don't wish the process of pulling a disgusting parasite from your butt on anyone, it was such a massive wake-up call. I was determined to do whatever it took to never go through that again.

I started doing my research. It didn't take long for me to make the connection between what I was putting in my body and what had come out of it in that shower. When we lived in New York, sushi was all the rage. We easily ate it five days a week. In the minds of the young and broke, it was the ideal lunch or dinner: cheap, low calorie, and quick. There was a general rule of thumb to not eat sushi at places that smelled bad, but when you're tight on funds, you tend to bend the rules.

While there are a lot of issues with raw fish and parasites, it wasn't necessarily the sushi that was the issue. It was the cleanliness of these places. We got our salads from Korean markets because again it was cheap, not clean. All the food we ate was at funky little places where cleanliness was not a priority. It's the New York way—the dingier the place, the better the food it's hiding. I once walked by one of my favorite restaurants late at night after it had closed. I will never forget the image of a huge rat making the tables, chairs, and countertops its playground. If camera phones had existed then, I would have had a viral video on my hands.

The truth is, we have no idea how clean restaurants are, even the ones that appear to be immaculate or have been lauded with the health code "A" rating. When Marc and I moved to Los Angeles, we had hundreds of dinners out at a (still) famous, nice sushi restaurant. That restaurant hung it's "A" rating with love and, especially for me, since I felt my parasite came from the sushi I was eating, it provided a lot of peace of mind. Years later, I met someone who worked for the health department who told me that the chef received his shining "A" in exchange for a huge load of cash. You just never know.

You're probably a bit grossed out and maybe even rescheduling that dinner date you have for Friday. In addition, you're probably wondering what parasites and something that came out of my butt has to do with cancer.

Parasites do two main bad things to our bodies, which can lead to cancer and/or seriously hurt someone battling cancer. **One,** parasites drain you of nutrients and produce cancer-causing wastes. So, even if you're loading your body with goodness, your parasite is eating them up. **Two,** they destroy your gut and digestive system and, as we learned in hack two, a gut that doesn't work sends everything haywire.

When parasites make a home for themselves in your body, they begin to feed off your cells, as well as the foods which you consume. Although they can cause a wide variety and range of ailments, the symptoms can be hard to detect. Symptoms can include cramps, brain fog, joint pain, diarrhea, gas, trouble falling asleep or staying asleep, rashes or hives, fatigue, depression, not feeling satiated after eating, anemia, and more. As you can tell, these are vague symptoms that can be attributed to a lot of other issues.

It's easy to acquire parasites while traveling abroad, eating contaminated food or water, or spending time with an infected animal. You might be thinking that because you never eat sushi or don't travel internationally that this is a chapter to skip, but those are just more common triggers. Studies have shown that up to 90 percent of people in North America suffer from at least one form of parasite, so hold tight.

I feel passionately about parasites because it's something that is often overlooked. When I give my clients a list of things to get checked out before their next appointment, getting checked for parasites is the number one thing that comes back unchecked. We don't think it's a priority and we also feel like if we had a parasite it would be really obvious: we'd feel terrible or weight would be falling off, but the truth is parasites can go undetected for a long time wreaking havoc on our insides.

It's funny—as I've been compiling research for this chapter I have heard multiple stories about people and parasites. One friend was sure his recent weight loss was due his new healthy eating and running regime, but couldn't explain his stomach issues. He went to a doctor who told him that the weight loss and stomach issues were both the product of a parasite, likely one he got while on a film set in Texas a month or two prior. Another friend posted on Facebook a video of the live, squirming parasite she found when she opened her package of fresh, organic, wild-caught salmon. Another friend was hospital-ridden for weeks with a parasite she assumed she had gotten from all her international travels, but doctors told her they actually think she picked it up from something she ate near her home in San Francisco. Three fairly big cases all coming to my attention within the last few days—this is not random, it's an epidemic.

I recommend getting checked for parasites every six months. Here's the tricky thing—we often check for parasites with stool tests but many parasites will die within one hour of being out of the body. Talk to your doctor about ensuring that your stool is checked immediately after coming out of the body to make sure your test doesn't falsely come back clean.

To get rid of my parasites, I had to go on a heavy-duty antibiotic for six weeks. Yuck! I'd love to have you avoid that, so here is how to combat the nasty parasite world:

Eat Clean

I can see the Amazon review now: "In every chapter, Goodman just told us to eat clean." Well that's because you should! This shouldn't surprise you, but a clean diet is key to making sure you aren't creating an inviting home for parasites. This will help you avoid getting them as well as clear out ones you might have.

Eating clean helps your body naturally eliminate parasites before they can do harm. If you are exposed to parasites and eat a poor diet, you will suffer much greater complications. Parasites breed on those who are nutrient deficient and thrive in that environment. Eating whole, organic foods and eliminating sugars, processed foods, gluten, and other inflammatory foods is the first step to a parasite-free body.

Eating clean reduces overall inflammation, boosts immune function, and helps you focus on eliminating parasites. Foods to avoid are: sugar, artificial sweeteners, wheat, dairy, fried foods, alcohol, caffeine, processed foods, deli meats, and any food that you have a sensitivity to.

If you do have parasites, there a few foods that they really hate, so stock up on the following:

- **Garlic**—when it comes to bacteria, parasites, cancer, and fungi, garlic has your back. Not only does it have the power to kill parasites, but it helps eliminate them from your body. Allicin, a powerful component found in garlic, boosts your immune system and fights infection. Allicin is most potent in fresh garlic, so it's best consumed raw. As long as you don't have a hot date coming up, you can eat a whole, raw clove. You can also chop it and add it to a glass of water or a smoothie. Not only can garlic kill preexisting parasites but it has the ability to prevent parasitic eggs from reaching the earliest stages of development, which will minimize parasite activity. Garlic can also help neutralize and eliminate harmful toxins left behind by parasites.

- **Pumpkin seeds**—Pumpkin seeds are a great snack. Although these seeds will not kill parasites, they will help flush them out. Compounds in pumpkin seeds paralyze parasites, so they cannot cling to your intestinal wall and are therefore flushed out. Either eat pumpkin seeds raw or on their own as a snack, or blend 200 grams with a cup of natural probiotic yogurt and a tablespoon of coconut oil (which is an antiparasitic food as well).

- **Coconut oil**—Coconut oil has antibacterial and antimicrobial properties.

- **Probiotic-rich foods**—Consuming high-probiotic foods that I talked about in the "gut" chapter can keep parasites in check and improve the health of the gut.

Increase Your Oxygen Intake

Oxygen helps promote healing and overall wellness. Both healthy cells and good bacteria are considered to be aerobic. Unlike parasites, which are anaerobic, healthy cells require oxygen to survive. Viruses, parasites, and pathogens all thrive in non-oxygenated environments. When you change the environment that parasites are currently living in, you will destroy them more easily.

If you live in a busy city, you will most certainly want to increase your oxygen intake. Smog and the burning of fossil fuels has lowered the average level of oxygen in the air. So, how can you increase your oxygen intake?

- **Food**—A balanced, raw-food diet can do wonders for your oxygen intake. Chlorophyll, which is found in dark leafy greens for instance, is high in oxygen as well as beneficial vitamins and minerals. When you consume more raw green juices and water, you will achieve a steady supply of oxygen.

- **Exercise**—Although food and water are great ways to increase your oxygen intake, exercise is also ideal. If possible, go for a walk, run or cycle in a heavily wooded area. Hiking trails are ideal for a nice afternoon stroll.

- **Yoga and meditation**—I practice both yoga and meditation, as they support the body and mind. Whether or not you take part in these practices as well, deep breathing is a must. When you take part in proper breathing techniques, you oxygenate your blood, which helps to detoxify your body.

- **Clean air**—In order to achieve the greatest deep-breathing benefits, clean, fresh air is a must. If you do live in a city area with high concentrations of smog, invest in an air filtration system. If you live in a more rural area, keep your windows open often, allowing for proper airflow.

- **House plants**—One of the easiest and most beautiful ways to increase oxygen levels in your home is to invest in a bunch of indoor plants. Plants increase oxygen and eliminate toxins in the air. For the best results, purchase two plants per 100 square feet. Some of the best options include, but are not limited to, English ivy, spider plants, aloe vera, Chinese evergreen, devil's ivy, and peace lilies.

Natural Supplements—Some of these supplements are the same as in the gut chapter.

There are some great natural supplements available, which can help detoxify your body and contribute to more positive health. Not only can supplements help boost functioning, but they also help reverse vitamin deficiencies. Remember, deficiencies and parasites go hand-in-hand.

- **Black walnut**—This has been used historically for the treatment of parasites.

- **Wormwood**—This perennial herb is a powerful remedy for intestinal worms. Both wormwood and black-walnut hulls are known to kill adult worms. Not only is this herb known to kill parasites, but it also is known for its ability to fight cancerous cells. Amazingly, a study published in *Life Sciences* in January 2005 found that when wormwood, or artemisinin, was combined with iron, it killed cancer cells, yet left healthy cells alone. This same approach has been used for thousands of years in China, in order to effectively target and cure malaria.

- **Oregano Oil**—(talked about in the "gut" chapter), oregano has antibacterial and antiparasitic effects.

- **Grapefruit seed extract**—(talked about in the "gut" chapter), GSE has antiparasitic effects.

- **Strong multivitamin**—If you do not believe you're consuming all the nutrients you require on a daily basis, a good quality vitamin could help. Since poor eating habits contribute to parasite infestation, a multivitamin can help you maintain good general health.

- **Enzyme supplements**—(talked about in the "gut" chapter), these help manage parasites. An enzyme supplement that contains hydrochloric acid helps break down your food. That way, partially undigested food isn't left for parasites to dine on within your digestive system. Also, parasites cannot thrive when normal levels of enzymes are present.

It's important to get parasites out of your body and take care of your gut. Parasites love it when your digestive enzymes and acids are low. A healthy gut means that you are creating this environment for foreign things to live in your body and cause mayhem in your immune system.

Increase Your Fiber Intake

Dietary fiber or roughage, which is only found in the cell walls of plant-based foods, is known to help prevent cancer. By consuming more fiber, you decrease your risk of toxic build-up. The best way to prevent an infestation of parasites is to take preventative measures.

Fiber is crucial within your diet, as it helps keep your colon clear. When there's a buildup of waste, parasites are more prone to make a nice home for themselves. Fiber helps to sweep your colon of toxins and can even help eliminate parasites from the walls of your digestive tract.

Based on the average American diet, most individuals are only consuming around 10 grams of fiber daily. Considering 30 to 35 grams is needed to maintain your health and reduce your risk of cancer, it's critical that you increase your fiber intake. If you are currently battling cancer, it is necessary to consume up to 50 grams of fiber. There are two types of dietary fiber: soluble and insoluble.

Although soluble sources of fiber are all highly beneficial for your health, insoluble fiber is most strongly linked to cancer prevention and waste removal. This includes wheat bran, barley, pinto beans, carrots, brown rice, broccoli, leafy greens, nuts, seeds, and more.

Sweat

As your body kills off parasites, their byproducts must be removed from the body, along with the toxins that they might have bound to. Some of these are best removed through the sweat glands, so let your body sweat by exercising and getting in hot tubs or saunas during the healing process. Also, soaking in an Epsom-salt bath (½ cup Epsom salt in hot bath water) will also help remove toxins through the skin.

elissa goodman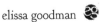

Cleanse Your Bowels

The best type of colon cleansers to kill parasites are those that first remove any blockages from the colon. Blockages arise from compacted fecal matter, which builds up when you do not have bowel movements on a regular basis. This leads to constipation and bloating. Once any blockages are removed from the colon, the cleanser can then easily eliminate the parasites.

If you're panicking thinking about the parasites crawling around inside of you—don't. Like all issues, there's a solution. These days, I am not a huge fan of colonics, as I think they are too harsh on the body. I prefer coffee enemas, a fabulous natural option if you have parasites. But I am grateful for the wakeup call my colonic provided. I, like most people today, did not consider parasites a threat nor did I ever think I could experience a huge one sharing my shower with me.

At the end of the day, I don't know if my parasite came from cheap sushi or a glass of water or someone's pet. We are a culture that eats out a lot, we socialize, we eat and drink stuff that, for the most part, we cannot trace its life path. The more we do that, the more parasites become a prevalent problem. When my clients come to me with digestive issues, it's my job to figure out if it's Candida, parasites, chemical overload, or something else. There is always an underlying base problem that's happening when we have a symptom.

It's a good reminder of how important it is to have a strong immune system and to be in tune to the way you are feeling. It's easy to chalk up symptoms to something else, but it's important to pay attention to what might be your body asking for backup.

Parasites are dangerous because they affect your ability to absorb nutrients, stop your body from being as healthy as possible, and ultimately open the floodgates to illness. Do parasites cause cancer? No. Can the effect they have on your body make your body a cancer-friendly environment. Absolutely. You have to provide the right environment for parasites to grow. If you create an unwelcome home—they won't live there.

Parasites to me, are the literal and metaphorical example that stuff is entering your body, living in your body, thriving in your body, changing your body, and affecting your body without your consent. So often we don't want to deal with stuff like this until it becomes an issue. We'll make time for that test if the symptoms are ruining our vacation plans and we'll cut out the dairy if it makes us too sick to walk, but not before that.

Let parasites be the little, silent reminder that you are in charge of taking care of your body **every day.** Not just on days you feel sick or days you want to look good. Every. Day. If my story isn't motivation enough to get checked and cleaned out, I don't know what is!

> *"I am in charge of my body and I lovingly take control of all that enters it."*

HACK 5:
Dirty Mouth

Did you know that more than 700 different strains of bacteria have been detected within the human mouth?

—Oral and Dental Health Resource Center

Did you know that silver fillings (also known as amalgams), are made up of mercury, a strong neurotoxin that can cause neurological issues, autoimmune issues, and cancer?

—Dr. Joseph Mercola, Mercola.com, September 2011

Did you know that bacteria can pass from your gums into your bloodstream, and oral pathogens make their way to distant parts of your anatomy, causing serious health problems?

—Dr. Joseph Mercola, Mercola.com, March 2014

One of the most common questions I get asked about my job is what my favorite part is. For me, there is nothing better than the sheer fact that I get to do this for a living. I had a passion and a dream and today it's a reality. How cool is that? But the other main thing that I love about this job is how much it evolves every day. Being a nutritionist is not about picking out ten safe foods to eat and sticking to them. Sure there are some general rules to guide you, but it's not really as simple as that.

One, we are all unique and our bodies need unique things. Two, our bodies are completely connected. My ideal nutrition plan can never be the same as your ideal nutrition plan because we don't have the same medical history, we haven't lived through the same traumas,

elissa goodman

and we don't share the same emotional and physical connection to everything. All of this matters. I say this time and time again, but you can eat kale morning, noon, and night and it won't matter if you can't look at the bigger picture.

You need to care for *your* body and its needs and that means the *whole* body and its needs. Everything from your gut to your pinky toe to your teeth matters when it comes to optimal health. If you're facing cancer, you need to take on all aspects of your health.

A few years ago, I wouldn't be talking to you about your teeth. I would have no idea that your teeth had anything to do with your health. But, alas, I've evolved. About three years ago, I went to hear a doctor speak at a fundraiser for cancer research. It was one of the most impactful lectures I have ever seen. The doctor came from an integrative cancer clinic in Rosarita Beach, Baja California, Mexico. He was presenting his research that linked root canals to breast cancer.

What he found was that when someone gets a root canal, they created a perfect breeding ground for microbes. These viruses, yeast, mold, fungus, and bacteria can easily get inside the root canal and set up a safe and comfortable home. Because no blood reaches the inside of the tooth, the immune system cannot kill any of these microbes.

He grew suspicious of root canals and their effect on our bodies. The doctor's research confirmed that 98 percent of the women who came to see him with breast cancer had one or more root canal teeth on the same meridian as the original breast cancer tumor. In his clinic, each of his patients saw a biological dentist to have their mouth cleaned up before any other treatment and, most important, had their root canal teeth removed. The women who had done this were there—they were all cancer-free or had been in remission for years.

If this study had the same effect on you that it has on me, your jaw is probably on the floor. Sure, I knew that you should keep your teeth healthy, visit your dentist regularly, and floss at least half of the amount of time that you tell your dentist you do, but did I think my teeth could give me cancer? No.

This lecture sent me on a tailspin—I was so curious about other connections between oral health and overall health. The research I found was astounding—study after study connecting these two worlds. And all these years, I thought keeping my teeth healthy just meant a pretty smile!

Here's what I found:

Oral Health and the Link to Overall Health

The condition of your gums, teeth, and mouth absolutely contributes to your overall health. Our mouths are full of bacteria, which is typically controlled and managed through daily brushing and flossing. When we do not take proper care of our oral health, however, infections and gum disease can arise. Before we jump into cancer and the ways in which oral health increases your risk, let's examine a few other diseases and conditions which can arise from poor oral health.

- **Cardiovascular disease**—It's believed that clogged arteries, heart disease, and stroke might be linked to poor oral health. Based on inflammation and infection, the bloodstream and heart become exposed to oral bacteria. More specifically, endocarditis occurs when there's an infection in the inner lining of your heart. Once again, bacteria from your mouth cause this, spreading throughout your body via your bloodstream.

- **Diabetes**—When you suffer from diabetes, you lose the ability for your body to fight infections at full force. This increases your risk of gum disease and oral infections. Diabetics need to take extra care of their gums and teeth, as these oral issues have been linked to poor glycemic control.

 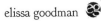

- **HPV**—Within recent years, scientists have uncovered the link between HPV (human papillomavirus) and cancer. Although HPV is typically known as a sexually transmitted disease, a 2013 study at the University of Texas linked poor oral health to an increased risk of contracting HPV.

  Within the University of Texas, 3,400 participants over the age of 30 were examined. Those who displayed poor oral hygiene had a 56 percent greater chance of being infected with HPV in comparison to those who had good oral health. Those who suffered from gum disease were at an even greater risk.

  HPV has been linked to cervical, vaginal, vulvar, and oral cancer. What researchers believe, is that when an individual suffers gum inflammation, sores, or ulcers, this provides an entry for HPV. As I mentioned earlier, lifestyle choices are what pull this kind of disease out from a dormant space, but it's still important to recognize the link.

Understanding the Link between Inflammation and Cancer

I talk about inflammation a lot and I want to be sure that you understand what I mean when I say that. Inflammation isn't just being bloated from a big meal or an allergic reaction. Our immune system is an incredible shield, protecting us each and every day. One of the key weapons of our immune system's defense is inflammation. To be fair, without inflammation, we more than likely wouldn't live past infancy. Inflammation is like your protective older brother—it's designed to remove harmful bacteria, chemicals. and even injured cells.

Sounds kind of nice, doesn't it? Well, inflammation tends to be a double-edged sword. Unfortunately, too much inflammation can severely impact your health. When you experience chronic inflammation, this is what leads to a number of diseases. So, how does something so beneficial, turn into cancer?

Inflammation doesn't necessarily create cancer, but it sure can fuel it. It's believed that when a small tumor begins to grow, it manages to survive from oxygen and nutrients within its immediate environment. Once it begins to grow, the demands for survival also increase. As the tumor grows, it releases chemical signals and immune cells begin to target and infiltrate. Once these immune cells are inside the tumor, they secrete small proteins called cytokines. This causes the growth of blood vessels, which carries in oxygen and nutrients.

So what's so bad about that? It gives the tumor the ability to access a much-needed blood supply and ignite cancer like fire. Inflammation can also encourage the spreading and further mutation of cancer cells. Scary.

Okay—so inflammation is bad, got it. But what does this have to do with oral health? Well, when you have poor oral hygiene, toxins and microorganisms circulate through your bloodstream, which can cause infections and chronic inflammation. Really scary.

Tons of research has shown that a bacterium commonly found in plaque has been linked to serious health concerns, specifically tumors within the colon. This bacterium triggers inflammation and activates cancer genes. Just as you have to address and handle the bacteria in your gut, you need to address and handle the bacteria in your mouth.

I once read about a study conducted in Sweden. Over a 24-year period (1985–2009) researchers examined the amount of plaque and poor oral hygiene in relation to premature death from cancer. A total of 1,390 young, healthy Swedes were randomly selected and each underwent oral examinations and were assessed in terms of socioeconomic status. They also took into account whether or not each person was a smoker.

The researcher hypothesized that poor oral health and hygiene was associated with an increased risk of cancer mortality and the results

 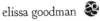

completely supported his thought. When he followed up with the participants, of the ones who had died, there was a significant difference in the amount of dental plaque they had.

While there are studies that cover extensive and lengthy amounts of time on this, this is still a fairly new topic in the nutrition world. I know as the chapters of this book pile up, you might be feeling a little overwhelmed with how many aspects of your life you need to worry about.

Remember, the best thing to do is to take this one day at a time without diminishing the importance of the whole. Baby steps toward a grander picture, where body, mind, and soul are all ready and willing to kick cancer's ass. Today, let's focus on some cancer-kicking teeth. It is essential to keep your mouth clean and, as more research emerges, it's clear that there's a distinct connection between the bacteria in your mouth and cancer.

Here are some strategies to improve oral health.

Consume a healthy diet

Just as a nutrient-dense diet helps balance your gut bacterial flora, it helps balance your oral bacterial flora. Following the nutritional guidelines I have laid out in this book and cutting out processed foods and sugar is step one to oral health. You can take it a step further by loading up on the fermented foods we talked about in the gut chapter. Options like kimchi, sauerkraut, and kefir provide beneficial bacteria and create a balanced oral environment.

Practice proper brushing and flossing

My dentist is going to love me for this! Brushing discipline has a lot to do with oral health care. Here are some tips on doing it right:

- **Floss regularly**—Ideally after each meal, realistically once a day. This reduces bacteria, which forms plaque between your teeth. It also removes buildup along your gum line, which leads to inflammation. Make sure you're buying a non-waxed floss.

- **Clean your toothbrush**—Once a week, soak your toothbrush in hydrogen peroxide. This is a safe and effective way to kill bacteria that accumulate and thrive on toothbrushes.

- **Cut the fluoride**—Do NOT use toothpaste with fluoride in it. Instead purchase an all-natural one or make your own. It's crazy easy to make one with coconut oil, baking soda, sea salt, and a few drops of organic peppermint essential oil.

- **Kill bacteria on your gums**—Make a mix of baking soda and salt and leave it on your gum line for about 15 minutes before rinsing. This will significantly reduce levels of plaque.

Try oil pulling

This practice has been around for thousands of years. When done effectively, you can pull toxins and bacteria out of your gums and mouth so that they do not spread through your body. Once a day, swish about a tablespoon of coconut oil around your mouth and through your teeth for about 15 minutes. When you're done, spit it out, and rinse. Do NOT swallow the oil or you will be swallowing a toxic soup.

Have your fillings checked

If you have suffered from any form of tooth decay, you more than likely have at least one silver filling. These silver fillings, also known as amalgams, have been used for more than a century with millions of people worldwide. These fillings are a mixture of metals, including liquid mercury. In fact, by weight, approximately 50 percent of silver fillings are this toxic element.

Unfortunately, these fillings can release mercury in the form of vapor. The vapor is absorbed by your organs and increases your risk of health complications. The greater your exposure is to mercury, the more your immune system, heart, lungs, and other organs are affected.

The main issue is that mercury is bio-accumulative, meaning that your body is absorbing toxic materials faster than it can eliminate them. Basically, toxins such as mercury accumulate in various tissues, gradually building up. Considering mercury is a known neurotoxin, causing chronic illness and autoimmune disorders, this is a major concern.

The government considers mercury to be a toxic waste, yet it is the most common material in dental fillings. Norway and Sweden have banned the use of mercury, but unfortunately the United States has been far too slow in terms of taking action. If you already have these silver fillings, you should reach out to a biological dentist. He or she will help you better understand whether or not your current fillings are toxic.

I understand that you trust those who are qualified and experienced within their position, but it's crucial that you question your dentist. If you're not comfortable with something, speak up. If you decide to have silver fillings removed, a dental rubber dam will be required. This will allow you to isolate the tooth, minimizing the amount of vapor being released. If you do require a cavity to be filled, ensure that porcelain or composite fillings are being used.

I have long felt that my exposure to mercury played into my cancer. I grew up on tuna fish sandwiches, as an adult I lived on sushi, and I had a mouth full of fillings. The effects of mercury toxicity in me were obvious in retrospect—I felt weak and tired and couldn't think. I had muscle pains and twitches, insomnia, digestive issues, food allergies, as well as bouts of depression and anxiety.

Once I slowly detoxified myself, I felt so much better. I have seen this over and over in my patients too. From chronic fatigue and fibromyalgia, to depression, anxiety, obesity, dementia, Parkinson's disease, cancer, heart failure, and heart disease, the message is clear—we are being poisoned!

Think twice before having a root canal

When David came home last year and announced his dentist told him he needed a root canal, I freaked out. Ever since hearing that doctor speak and doing my own research, having a root canal is like taking on a smoking habit in my book. When you have a root canal, the tooth essentially dies and is cut-off from the regular blood supply. Within our teeth, there are many little tubules, which remain after the root canal is complete. Microscopic organisms within these tubules no longer gain the oxygen and nutrients required, so they transform into toxins and bacteria.

Once your immune system weakens for any reason, your body will not target and destroy the bacteria that leak from this dead tooth. Bacteria then find their way into the bloodstream where they can thrive in other tissues, glands, or organs. This can lead to cancer.

Here's the bummer. Our options are limited, and if you've ever had a root canal you know that it's not exactly something you can avoid. You do have the option to remove the tooth completely and have an implant put in, but that is a bit drastic. The best thing you can do here is keep your body healthy and your immune system strong. If bacteria hit the bloodstream, you want to know your body can fight them before they become a problem.

Don't be so quick to remove your wisdom teeth

Similar to root canals, I wish wisdom teeth surgery was something that just didn't exist in the world. It's been reported that up to 67 percent of wisdom teeth extractions are unnecessary and they have become so second nature, oftentimes dentists recommend removal just because you've reached a certain age. The problem is, once they are removed, they often leave big sockets that rarely heal.

elissa goodman

These sockets can fill with bacteria, causing infection and further inflammation. Dentists can fail to remove all the connective tissue from the socket, which can lead to cavitation—tiny bony holes.

Much like the root canals, options are limited. If you have to get them removed because of a problem, that's one thing, but don't be so quick to have them removed just because. At the end of the day, knowledge is power. It's not always about having an alternative as it's about preparing yourself, understanding what's happening, and being aware that there are consequences to actions even if they are taken in the spirit of good health. I also highly recommend consulting a biological dentist with any concerns.

Extra Helpful Information

What You Need to Know about Chemotherapy and Your Mouth

If you or a loved one is currently undergoing chemotherapy and radiation, you will notice side effects and changes within your body. Some of these issues are directly experienced within your mouth. Since chemotherapy uses drugs that kill cancer cells, normal healthy cells are also affected.

In your mouth, you might experience noticeable issues with your gums, teeth, and even your saliva. This increases your risk of oral infection, which will not benefit your current treatment. Typically, these side effects surface during chemotherapy when one's oral health was poor to begin with.

If you are going to start chemotherapy, visit your dentist at least a month prior, if possible. If you have already begun treatment, visit your dentist immediately (consider a holistic dentist). During any cancer treatment, you need to focus on properly caring for your mouth and oral health.

In order to avoid complications, you should focus on some key areas regarding your oral health. Cancer treatment will require you to take extra caution, as you continue to support your overall health.

The following suggestions will help you prevent sores and infection during cancer treatment:

1. **Hydration**—Every single cell in your body requires water so proper hydration is essential for anyone, but especially those undergoing cancer treatment. Without proper hydration, your body cannot function efficiently. Due to the side effects of chemotherapy and other cancer treatments, if you are undergoing these treatments your risk of dehydration skyrockets. Make sure you are drinking half your bodyweight in water every day at a minimum.

   In order to increase the level of moisture within your immediate environment, use a humidifier. This will help maintain a moist mouth and throat. When you continually moisturize wounds, you enable them to heal faster. A recent study found that cancer patients, who utilized a humidifier daily during radiation treatment, experienced nearly 50 percent fewer visits to the hospital based on their treatment's side effects.

2. **Increase saliva production**—During radiation or chemotherapy, many individuals will experience dry mouth. This typically occurs because the salivary glands are not producing enough saliva to keep their mouth moist and healthy. Not only does it aid in chewing, tasting, and swallowing, but saliva also helps your mouth maintain the right balance of bacteria.

   When there isn't any saliva in your mouth, bacteria are able to grow more rapidly. Unfortunately, this can lead to infections or sores, as well as cavities and gum disease over time. Depending on where radiation therapy is directed on your body, you could potentially experience long-term dry mouth. However, most individuals notice their symptoms subside two to eight weeks after radiation treatment has ended.

Although a lack of saliva cannot be prevented, it can be managed and controlled. One of the easiest ways is to regularly chew gum (especially xylitol-containing gum) or suck on all-natural candy.

Sonic brushing is another area that can help aid in more positive oral health. Amazingly, these toothbrushes can vibrate at more than 30,000 brush strokes per minute. This, of course, helps clean hard-to-reach areas and remove more bacteria. Sonic brushing also encourages fluid dynamics, due to the intense vibrational speed it provides. The fluids that are within your water at the time of brushing (water and saliva) start to move rapidly, damaging plaque colonies. This helps reach areas where your brush simply can't. Basically, the intensity of the sonic brush causes water and saliva to propel against the surface of your teeth.

If you are receiving radiation, acupuncture could help you increase saliva production, while minimizing pain. Perhaps you have completed treatment, yet you're still suffering from the effects of dry mouth (this is especially common for those who received radiation directly to their head or neck).

Based on a study conducted at the University of Texas MD Anderson Cancer Center, researchers reported that when given two acupuncture treatments for four weeks, symptoms of dry mouth significantly improved.

3. **Prevent cavities**—When I was a kid, my biggest fear was that I would go to the dentist and he would tell me I had a cavity—well, some things never change! Cavities are signs of tooth decay. This can lead to worse oral health, as well as pain. It's essential that you keep your mouth clean, so that cavities do not develop before, during, or after treatment. The majority of oral health concerns are preventable.

You must cut out sugar, because when sugar is combined with bacteria in your mouth, it turns into plaque. Once plaque builds up, small holes can begin to form in your teeth. This is the beginning stage of a cavity. If left untreated, bacteria and plaque can reach your nerves and blood vessels once the hole has eroded past your tooth enamel. This, of course, causes pain and possible infections.

Although sugar is the main culprit in terms of tooth decay (based on the bacteria it interacts with), you can effectively intervene by brushing and flossing often. Since fluoride accumulates in the body, choose all-natural toothpaste that does NOT contain this mineral.

I also highly suggest a tongue scraper, as it's noninvasive, yet effective. If you have ever noticed a white-yellowish layer on your tongue, that's bacteria, dead cells, toxins, and food. Isn't that appetizing and lovely? If you would like to reduce this build-up, a tongue scraper is a great solution. This simple cleansing practice is widely used in both the holistic and Eastern worlds. You simply scrap this layer off your tongue, which removes the soft plaque that can lead to cavities and tooth decay.

4. **Prevent soft tissue injury and infection**—Cancer treatment, especially radiation and chemotherapy, can lead to open sores. Although you cannot always prevent soft tissue injuries, you can take a couple of proactive measures to reduce the severity, as well as the duration. This will not only provide you with relief, but could help prevent infection and further oral complications.

   Chemotherapy, for instance, is used to kill rapidly growing cells, such as cancerous cells. Since some healthy cells rapidly divide and grow as well, chemotherapy and radiation can also threaten these cells. The cells that line the inside of your mouth are a prime example of these rapidly growing, healthy cells. Chemotherapy massively diminishes your immune system, which allows bacteria and viruses to thrive.

As mentioned, there is no guarantee that you will prevent sores and ulcers, but you can reduce your risk. When you visit your dentist before (or during) treatment, discuss the risks associated with cancer treatment and mouth sores. If you haven't already, immediately quit smoking, develop a strong oral health routine, and focus on a nutrient-rich diet.

It has been found that individuals who are deficient in iron, folic acid, or vitamin B12 tend to develop canker sores and lesions more often. If you are prone to ulcers and sores, it's important to boost your immune system. Two B-vitamins in particular, vitamin B9 (folic acid) and vitamin B1 (thiamine), as well as vitamin C and zinc will help prevent and heal ulcers.

It's also important to note that stress is a trigger for many people. If stress is potentially causing sores to develop in your mouth, take this time to begin more stress-minimizing activities, such as walking daily, meditation, or yoga. This will not only benefit your oral health, but your whole body and mind. Another reason to do yoga? What's not to love?

We all grow up learning that brushing our teeth is a part of good hygiene. It's one of the first things we do to take care of ourselves—before we can shower by ourselves or wash our hands, before we are potty-trained, we have a toothbrush in our mouths. Unlike potentially taking a fast-food diet and turning it toward a whole-foods diet, this isn't about doing a total 180.

Proper and holistic oral hygiene is about education, consistency, and choosing the right products. In the few extra minutes each week that it would take you to make a fluoride-free toothpaste and floss your teeth, you could save your life. This is also an important lesson in not always trusting every medical professional in your life. Just because someone has a degree does not mean they know what's best for you. Neither do I! Only you know what's best for you. Have I said this enough yet? ☺ Now brush your teeth!

> *"My body is a powerful temple and I encourage each part of it to be filled with life and energy."*

HACK 6:
Toxic Buildup

Did you know the average newborn baby has 287 known toxins in his or her umbilical cord blood?

—Dr. Mark Hyman, drhyman.com, May 2013

Did you know you are exposed to an average of 2,100,000 toxins each and every day?

—Global Healing Center, December 2013

Did you know this means you are exposed to 2.5 billion pounds of toxic chemicals and 6 million pounds of mercury each year?

—Dr. Hyman, drhyman.com, May 2013

"By cleansing your body on a regular basis and eliminating as many toxins as possible from your environment, your body can begin to heal itself, prevent disease, and become stronger and more resilient than you ever dreamed possible."

—Dr. Edward Group III, CEO of Global Healing Center, January 2015

I have a client who came to me because he was so mentally and physically fatigued, and he had digestion issues, high cholesterol, and liver problems. He looked and seemed like a healthy guy and his issue was not immediately transparent. I started asking him about his work. He worked in the produce business and he was constantly visiting farms and evaluating all types of produce.

 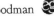

I had a feeling he might be overexposed to chemicals the farmers spray on produce.

I had him get his blood tested and it came back with a high amount of chemicals. He could not believe it—for the most part, what he ate was healthy and thanks to his work he always had tons of fresh vegetables in the house. But the vegetables he was selling were not organic so he was exposed to lots of chemicals.

People assume toxins can only enter your body through your mouth, but your skin is the largest organ and is constantly absorbing everything it comes into contact with. From birth until now, your body has become a toxic waste dump and now that you are ready to make a change, you must start by facing this dirty truth. Your body is drowning in cancer-causing toxins that must be removed. We are exposed to toxins every day, many of which remain in our bodies.

When toxins enter your body, your natural, healthy alkaline state is converted to an acidic state, where acid eats away at practically every organ in your body. In this state, your body becomes an inviting breeding ground for cancer. This stress weakens the immune system and increases susceptibility to disease, viruses, and infections.

Toxins bombard and invade you from all angles: your food, water, environment, prescription medications, cleaning products, soaps, lotions, perfumes, and even chemicals that are used to manufacture your food and clean your house, all play a role.

One of the scariest forces in all of this is Monsanto. You might have heard a little or a lot about this agricultural corporation, which was one of the first companies to combine agriculture with biotechnology. There is a lot of controversy around these guys and it is well-deserved. What they are doing is downright scary. The man who invented these toxins is a long-time pharmaceutical industry veteran who knows a lot about additives, toxins, and quick fixes. Both of these industries are huge moneymakers, which is scary for the consumer.

elissa goodman

With Monsanto, it has found success in manufacturing dangerous herbicides and genetically modified crops. Remember Agent Orange? That was a Monsanto product, which exposed up to 4.5 million Vietnamese civilians and 2.8 million US soldiers. It was tied to cancer, Parkinson's, diabetes, spinal bifida, reproductive abnormalities, and developmental disabilities in children. Monsanto's newest herbicide, Roundup, is one of the world's most widely used weed killers. Chances are high that the produce you eat has been exposed to Roundup. The active ingredient in Roundup is glyphosate, which is carcinogenic to humans and has been linked to issues such as Parkinson's and fatal kidney disease. This is so scary to me and I hope it is a bit of wake-up call for you.

The importance of eating a whole, nutrient-dense diet like we discussed in the past chapters is the foundation for clearing toxins out of your body. Our bodies were not created to process what are now staples in the American diet. When foods are not natural, like processed and sugary foods, our bodies do not know how to break those chemicals down. Instead, chronic inflammation occurs and chronic inflammation to cancer is the beautiful home, with the welcome mat and a warm meal waiting inside. Cancer loves inflammation.

Ask your grocer where the produce comes from. Monsanto and the millions of other companies like it, thrive on ignorance. We need to stop being afraid to ask questions that relate to our own health and wellbeing.

Taking control of your diet is unfortunately just the beginning of getting rid of that toxic buildup. You cannot totally control all the toxins in the air, but you can limit your exposure by what you eat and put on your body.

You do not have to be a farmer or run a produce company to have direct exposure to these chemicals. They are everywhere. It is important to be continually detoxing to limit the chemicals that can make a home in your organs and tissues. If you are constantly throwing out the trash, you are way ahead of others who allow the trash to pile up.

Here are my favorite detoxing tricks.

Try an Infrared Sweat

When I had cancer, I frequently visited a spa called Beverly Hot Springs. I never felt guilty about spending hours there, because I knew it was helping me heal from my cancer. The balmy waters of the Beverly Hot Springs gush from a natural artesian well 2,200 feet beneath the Earth's surface. The water is heated by geothermal heat, essentially heat from the Earth's interior and contains minerals and elements such as alkaline, radium, sulfur, sodium, and alkaline sodium chloride, which have lots of healing properties and health benefits.

Nowadays, I'm a bit too busy to be soaking in a spa for hours. Luckily four years ago, I discovered infrared sweating. Infrared heat penetrates the organs so they start to sweat out the toxins. There is a special place in Los Angeles called the Shape House, an urban sweat lodge that I go to for an hour and leave feeling like a new person. The sweating is deep and profuse yet the temperature is lower than traditional saunas so it is great for those of you who do not love the heat.

If you do not have an infrared sauna near you, a traditional sauna is still great. You can also buy infrared blankets online which are incredible. Hot yoga also induces detoxification. Any kind of sweating will help promote opening the pores and letting the toxins out.

With that being said, there is a difference between sweating from a hard, cardio workout and sweating in a sauna. Cardio is good for the heart but to get the detoxification benefits, you have to go to the deeper level where you are heating your body to the place in

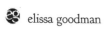

which your organs are sweating. The steam heat that you find in saunas opens your pores and allows for a greater level of tolerance. For example, you would benefit from spending twenty minutes in a 140-degree sauna, but you would not benefit from spending twenty minutes in a 100-degree house. Moral of the story: get your sweat on!

Detox Bath

I mentioned this in an earlier chapter but it is such an incredible tool for those who do not have access to any kind of sauna, and it's super simple and effective. Run the water in your bath as hot as you can stand it and add in 1 cup of Epsom salt, 2 cups of baking soda, and a few drops of lavender essential oil. Soak in there for at least 30 minutes. The Epsom salt and baking soda help pull toxins out from your skin and the lavender will induce a total state of relaxation. You will be shocked at how much you are sweating.

In fact, you need to be careful. Once you are done with your soak, take caution when standing up. You will have lost so many toxins you might actually feel a little lightheaded. I recommend hydrating before, during, and after!

Drink a Green Juice or Smoothie Every Day

When I got diagnosed with cancer, I began drinking raw juices like crazy. But my options were limited at stores and I did not see home juicers for sale. I drank a lot of carrot juice and other simple stuff: spinach and beet or cucumber juices. At the time, it was not hip or cool to drink juices and once I had recovered from my cancer I lost the habit.

After Marc died, I remember thinking, "Oh, shit. My daughters now have two parents with cancer, one of which did not make it. I have to get back to taking care of myself because I have to be here for them." It is so easy to do the right things when you're pushed against a wall, but what I am trying to stress is that we need to do the right things today and every day. No matter what, do not wait until you are in a bad situation to start taking care of yourself.

I got back into juicing and now I hardly go a day without it. There is no feeling quite like drinking a green juice. You can truly feel the influx of goodness immediately into your body. How could you not love that feeling?

Green juice is more than just a huge dose of veggies, the natural chlorophyll actually helps push toxins out of your fat stores and provides you with an abundance of enzymes, vitamins, minerals, and phytochemicals.

A lot of people ask me if they can have a green smoothie instead of a juice. In my world, nothing beats a juice. It is so nutrient dense and allows you to consume a larger amount of vegetables than you would normally. You probably would not eat six cucumbers, but juicing six cucumbers is easy. With that being said, the smoothie and the juice are both great.

Juice is more concentrated but a lot of people find smoothies to be an easier and a more convenient option. Smoothies allow you to be able to use frozen produce as opposed to constantly needing fresh produce in the house for a juice, and I understand that multiple trips to the grocery store in a week are not always that easy.

The main difference is that blended smoothies keep the fiber of the fruits and vegetables in, which slows the process of the food hitting your bloodstream. In juices, the fiber is removed so it is a direct hit to your bloodstream and into your cells.

At the end of the day, I care about you getting those vegetables in wherever and however you can. So if it is a juice or a smoothie, I'm happy. Just don't buy any of that store-bought crap! Those are loaded with sugars, preservatives, and other chemicals. Juices and smoothies are meant to be drunk when they are made, not to have any shelf life. Make your juices or smoothies at home and drink them right away. After 24 hours, their nutrients are super depleted.

Start Your Day with Water and Lemon

I love this detox trick because it is so easy and accessible. There is no excuse not to try this one! Warm water with lemon serves as the perfect "good morning drink," as it aids the digestive system in making the process of eliminating waste products from the body easier. It also helps with constipation, diarrhea, and ensuring smooth bowel functions.

Ideally, you continue to drink lemon water throughout the day. Bring a baggie of sliced lemons to work with you and pop a slice in every time you fill your water container. This will also help you make sure you are drinking enough water. Being properly hydrated prevents adrenal fatigue. When the body is fatigued, it cannot properly function and it leads to toxic buildup.

Lemon is incredible because it is high in vitamin C, which helps the liver process and eliminate toxins, but lime is almost equally as great so feel free to switch it up.

I like warm water or room temperature water. Steer clear of icy cold water; your body is forced to use energy to get that water to match its natural body temperature. This takes away energy that could be used for digestion.

Remember, you should be drinking a minimum of half your body weight in ounces each day in water. While you are at it, throw some lemon in it and get those toxins out of you!

Cleanse Your House

My clients are always willing to let me into their kitchens, but when I try to get into their bathrooms, closets, and laundry rooms they are bit more hesitant. I know it is overwhelming to acknowledge the chemicals in all our cleaning products, lotions, makeup, plastic containers, etc., but it is equally as important to address these items for their content.

Trust me, this is a really hard area for me. It is easy to see how pizza and cheeseburgers make you look bad. Bed linens? Perfumes? Anti-aging skin creams? They make you feel better. Long term, however, they can be lethal.

The best rule of thumb is to never use any product that you would not eat. Anything your skin is exposed to, your organs and insides are exposed to. Think about a nicotine patch. Why does that work? Because what you put on your skin goes directly to your bloodstream.

Luckily, the demand for natural products means there are tons of natural options on the market today. Look for products that use olive oil, coconut oil, aloe vera, charcoal, or other natural ingredients as a base. But beware! Don't just buy something because it's labeled as natural or organic. Environmental Working Group has a sensational website at that allows you to check all your household products for toxin levels. Spend an hour researching the products you use. They also have an incredible app that has changed my life. You can scan any product and it will give you its ranking and suggest better alternatives. It's a lifesaver when you're at the store. It's one of those perfect tools that can truly be the difference between this lifestyle being simple or complicated. I highly recommend utilizing their resources.

The amount of toxins we taken in daily through products is daunting. From the dryer sheets leftover on your sheets when you wake up in the morning, the plastic cup you drink water from, the soap you use in the shower, the chemical-laden toothpaste, the lotion you put on your body, the detergent remains on your towels and clothes, the toxic nonstick pan you cook your eggs in—the list goes on and on and we are not even through breakfast. Ah!

I will talk more about toiletries and makeup in the next chapter, but making your whole house a cancer-free zone is important. For example, did you know that nonstick pans contain toxins that after four years of being in your body are only decreased by half? Replace your cookware with cast iron, ceramic, or glass options.

elissa goodman

We do not have total control of all the chemicals and toxins we are exposed to, but we should take care of the ones we do have control over. I know this can seem like a huge undertaking. Here is my advice: start with products you use in the shower. These are the biggest threat because you use them while your pores have been opened from the hot water. Your body is just slurping these toxins up.

Then, the priority should be products that have prolonged exposure to you once you use them, such as cleaning supplies that stay on your countertops, lotions that sit on your body, and the cookware that leaves toxins on all your meals.

The last priority should be items you have shorter or limited exposure to, such as makeup you take off at the end of the day, nail polish remover that you do not use often, etc. I know it can be overwhelming so pick your battles wisely. The best example I can think of is nail polish versus nail polish remover. Both are loaded with toxins and should be avoided. But with nail polish remover you have a short exposure, whereas nail polish sits on your nails for a week or two, soaking those toxins in.

I know this is a lot to take in. Try taking it room by room. As with all of this, there is a bit of work to adapt to a better lifestyle, but once it is a part of your routine it will come so naturally to you. I used to feel so overwhelmed by changing out products in my home. But I started digging around online for some simple swaps. The first one I did was to make a white vinegar, water, and tea tree oil spray to replace most my cleaning products. It worked (and smelled!) better than what I using previously. Then I let coconut oil take over my bathroom routine and I feel totally in love! I now use it in place of makeup remover and lotion. I've even converted to using apple cider vinegar instead of deodorant. Trust me, if I can make these changes anyone can. The truth is, besides being much cheaper, they are actually simpler alternatives. The list goes on and on for healthy swaps you can make inside the home. I highly encourage you to spend a few minutes looking up some holistic alternatives for your most toxic products and let yourself be surprised at how much better they work!

You can also turn to the kitchen and incorporate some naturally detoxifying foods. Here are my favorites:

Detox Foods

Cilantro

The leaves of the coriander plant possess remarkable detoxifying abilities. Studies have shown that cilantro binds to heavy metals in the bloodstream, thereby purifying tissues, organs, and blood. Cilantro is able to attach to metals.

Parsley

Parsley helps eliminate salt that has built up in the kidneys, thereby purging the body of accumulated poisons like mercury, cadmium, and lead.

Wild blueberries (only from Maine)

They can draw heavy metals out from your brain. Also, they heal and repair any gaps created when heavy metals are removed, which is important for your brain tissue.

Atlantic dulse

It can bind to metals and cross the blood-brain barrier. It can go into deep hidden places of the body looking for mercury, binding to it, and never releasing it until it leaves the body.

Detox Supplements

We all need to be detoxing all the time to combat the chemicals we are constantly exposed to. Adding in any and all of the methods above, combined with a nutrient-rich diet, is a huge step toward getting rid of those chemicals. With that said, if you are someone like my client who had tons of chemical exposure through his job, I definitely recommend taking it up a level.

There are a few products I rely on for serious detoxing:

Barley Grass Juice Extract Powder

It can draw out heavy metals from your spleen, intestinal tract, pancreas, and reproductive system. It prepares the metals for complete absorption by the spirulina.

Spirulina (preferably from Hawaii)

It draws out metals from your nervous system and liver and absorbs heavy metals extracted by the Barley Grass Juice Extract Powder.

Zeolite

It has molecules (naturally occurring minerals, typically found in rocks and clay) that contain a powerful magnetic energy to pull the metals out of tissues and then pass them out of the body through urination and defecation.

I talk a bit more about these products in Appendix 3. They are super safe and even if you do not think you have been exposed to a lot of toxins you could still add them to your regular routine.

My intuition told me that treating my toxic cancer with toxic drugs seemed ignorant. Cancer drugs are notoriously noxious and come with devastating, and often lethal side effects. The pharmaceutical world is so desperate to give the illusion that it is fighting the good

elissa goodman

fight that many of these drugs are used despite the fact that they are not doing anything to improve the life of those diagnosed with cancer. In fact, they might be making it worse.

The best-selling (and extremely expensive) cancer drug Avastin, for example, was just recently phased out as a treatment for metastatic breast cancer after studies showed its dangerous side effects were far outweighed by its benefits.

Extra Helpful Information

My Tips for Lowering Your Risk of Chemical Exposure

- As much as possible, purchase organic produce and hormone-free foods to reduce your exposure to pesticides, growth hormones, GMOs, and synthetic fertilizers.
- Rather than using conventional or farm-raised fish, which are often heavily contaminated with PCBs and mercury, supplement with a high-quality purified fish oil or eat fish that is wild-caught and lab tested for purity.
- Eat mostly raw fresh foods, steering clear of processed, prepackaged foods of all kinds. This way you automatically avoid artificial food additives, including dangerous artificial sweeteners, food coloring, and MSG.
- Store your food and beverages in glass rather than plastic, and avoid using plastic wrap and canned foods (which are often lined with BPA- and BPS-containing liners).
- Have your tap water tested and, if contaminants are found, install an appropriate water filter on all your faucets (even those in your shower or bath).
- Only use natural cleaning products in your home.
- Switch to natural brands of toiletries such as shampoo, toothpaste, antiperspirants, and cosmetics.

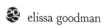

- Avoid using artificial air fresheners, dryer sheets, fabric softeners, or other synthetic fragrances.
- Replace your nonstick pots and pans with ceramic or glass cookware.
- When redoing your home, look for "green," chemical-free alternatives in lieu of regular paint and vinyl floor coverings.
- Replace your vinyl shower curtain with one made of fabric, or install a glass shower door. Most flexible plastics, like shower curtains, contain dangerous plasticizers like phthalates.
- Limit your use of drugs (prescription and over-the-counter) as much as possible. Drugs are chemicals too, and they will leave residues and accumulate in your body over time.
- Avoid spraying pesticides around your home or insect repellants that contain DEET on your body. There are safe, effective, and natural alternatives available.

I know sometimes it can feel like you cannot win—like everything has chemicals in it or everything is bad for you. I get it, it is exhausting and every day new studies come out proving that something else we use in our routine life is bad for us. It is so easy to get overwhelmed and not know where to start and to just give up before you have started trying. But you can do this and it is important.

Give yourself a realistic goal—"I'm going to redo one room a week and within six months I want to be totally natural." Rome was not built in a day and neither is your healthy lifestyle. But make it a priority to make baby steps, starting today.

"I am amazed at my body's ability to release and heal."

HACK 7:
Denial and the Suppression of Emotions

Did you know that 85 percent of all diseases are linked to an emotional element?

—US Centers for Disease Control and Prevention, February 2010

Did you know that suppressed emotions could increase your risk of heart disease by 47 percent and your risk of cancer by 70 percent?

—Harvard School of Public Health, September 2013

Did you know that yoga was first practiced in India more than 5,000 years ago, making it the oldest mind-body health system in existence?

—American Cancer Society, cancer.org

We are in an interesting time in our health culture. I firmly believe that many years from now, we will look back and see what a turning point this era has been. I touched on this a little bit earlier in the book, but we are coming out of an era of fad dieting. It's easy for me to see how the nutritional lifestyle I talk about here could be considered just another fad or quick fix. But instead, it's a return to basics.

The fads aren't working. The chemicals we are making food out of so that they lack calories are killing us. We are overweight, exhausted, and disease-ridden and we need a new answer. Slowly

 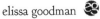

but surely, we are realizing that we need to cut the crap out and return to a place where vegetables are royalty and farmers are king. We are taking our food out of the microwave and onto the stove. We are honoring the difference between a salad with fried chicken and ranch dressing and a salad with raw veggies and olive oil. This, is progress. And this, is important.

But it's not all about what you eat. The way we live is equally, if not more, important. More often than having clients who eat tons of crap, I have clients who eat really well and can't figure out why they still feel like crap. I want to start exploring with you the other side to all of this besides what you eat.

Positive health comes from optimal physical and emotional and mental health. In order to get healthy, you have to nurture all areas of your health and wellbeing. We live in a culture where being strong and marching on is celebrated. We often wear our battle wounds, but not our journey, with pride. Suppressing our feelings is natural. Carry on. March on. Move on.

I believe that for many of us, we have, without even knowing it, learned how to suppress and deny our emotions. It's a natural coping mechanism that allows us to adjust to a new reality. Often it's easier to suppress our emotions than face the truth head-on. This can only protect us short term; in the long run it hurts us immensely. If you or a loved one has been diagnosed with cancer, you might be suppressing the emotions of that diagnosis. It's our body's instinct to take what is overwhelming and try to break it down and store it.

This cancer hack is incredibly important to me, because it's one of the biggest lessons I've learned in my experience. I have been suppressing emotions my entire life. There is no doubt in my mind that suppressing my emotions had a huge impact on me getting cancer. I grew up thinking that I couldn't trust anyone and that life was full of punches. I was taught that my feelings didn't matter, that love was conditional, and if I wanted love or respect, I better work overtime to earn it.

My parents are tough people who don't show a lot of emotion. My mom inherited her family's long history of trust issues. When she and my dad had success in their business, I think this sparked a lot of those issues in her. She was always self-conscious and wary of why people wanted to have a relationship with them. She started believing that everyone wanted to take advantage of them and had a hard time being honest.

My dad, on the other hand, was too trusting. I think she overcompensated for him and I saw both sides of the spectrum as being potentially dangerous. I was naturally really trusting, like my dad, but watching my mom, I began to question if blindly trusting people was the right thing to do. I started to not feel like I could trust my own instincts. I was incredibly sensitive and I didn't know how to be the emotionless person I thought my family wanted me to be. In the back of my mind I had this default setting of life sucks, people suck, and I suck. I was angry but anger wasn't something that was expressed in my house so I suppressed it.

Looking back there's no doubt in my mind that that outlook and suppressing that anger weakened me and made me susceptible to illness. In a weird way, I was waiting for something to come. Just another blow, right?

When I got diagnosed with cancer, I continued to beat myself up. I felt sad and helpless. I felt like I needed to just grin and bear it. I felt like I had to tell everyone else I was fine and it was going to be okay even though my insides were going a mile a minute. One day, I hit a breaking point. This was more than I could handle. This was more than I could suppress. I hit a wall and it felt like every emotion I had every suppressed had exploded in front of me. It was scary and messy but for the first time in my life, I really allowed myself to feel anger and grief and jealousy and fear and shame and guilt and doubt.

I thank my cancer every day for that wakeup call; that was the moment I started to find my own voice. That was just the beginning and many years of seeing a therapist, meditating, and yoga, and

elissa goodman

sometimes I still feel like I'm on the path of relearning how to feel and express myself. But I'm a million times better than I was before. I finally realized that the way we feel is part of being human, it's how we learn and grow and open up.

If you repress, deny, or run from your feelings, they will own you. They will chase you down again and again. In many negative forms they will arise and for those of you wondering if your cancer is one of those forms, I firmly believe that it's definitely possible.

I'm not going to ask you to march on, carry on, or move on. I'm not going to ask you to be a warrior right now. I'm going to ask you to be human. I know what it feels like to suppress emotions to a point where you don't even know that you are suppressing them. Relax and take a deep breath. We aren't going to rip open all your emotional wounds, but we aren't going to bandage them either. We are simply going to take one step forward, away from fear and toward emotion.

How Emotions Are Linked to Cancer

We have discussed a lot about diet and the ways our lifestyles contribute to an increased risk of cancer. Although your physical health is, of course, a vital piece of the cancer puzzle, your emotional health also plays a critical role. Eastern medicine believes that the emotions we carry apply directly to the body. When you carry around resentment and anger, for instance, these feelings directly threaten your immune system. We hold grief in our lungs, anger in our hearts, anxiety in our spleen, and so on. On top of that, when you do not deal with negative emotions, this can lead to an increase in stress hormones, such as cortisol.

Long term, these hormones are what create the link between your emotions and poor immune function, increasing your risk of cancer. This also plays a role during cancer treatment, as repressed negative emotions will continually affect your immune system, which, in turn, hinders your ability to fight the disease itself.

For those who develop cancer, it's typically due to a combination of both psychological and physiological factors. Just as poor nutrition and toxins can play a role, so can stress, lack of sleep, and emotional trauma. Does a stressful life automatically mean that you'll develop cancer? No, not exactly, but it can increase your risk based on additional factors.

If you're someone who has spent any of your life not dealing with your emotional health, getting a cancer diagnosis for yourself or a loved one is not going to be easily processed. It's completely normal to experience fear, anger, depression, sadness, resentment, and other emotions as the development of any illness is incredibly traumatic. It's incredibly important that you feel your feelings during this process.

Here are two areas to focus on when opening yourself up during this process.

Mindfulness

The idea of utilizing mindfulness-based interventions has become increasingly popular within cancer treatment. Within everyday life, we tend to focus on things we could have done differently; and what we can expect from the future, as we worry and plan. Mindfulness helps control our mental awareness, as we truly experience the present moment.

Whether you take part in mindfulness through deep meditation or not, you can take part in this beneficial practice by simply remembering to be present. Live in the moment, truly experiencing your surroundings. It's crucial that you stay in the moment during this process. Spending time focusing on the past or future is useless and can hurt your healing process. You cannot change the past; you cannot control the future. Mindfulness helps remind you that *you* are in charge of today. You are going to do the best you can, today. And when today is over, it's over. And you will do the best you can tomorrow.

If you aren't diagnosed, before cancer even has a chance to develop, you can implement positive strategies into your life. Mindfulness can be a proactive measure you can take, protecting your immune system and wellbeing. By improving your overall wellbeing, you will help prevent cancer, along with many other chronic conditions.

We live in a society where stress is all around us. Our jobs create an immense amount of stress, which tends to consume us. When you are stressed, your immune system is comprised and this can lead to a greater likelihood that you'll fall ill. In order to combat stress, mindfulness is a remarkable tool. It helps improve so many aspects of your life, as you increase mental focus, enjoy each and every experience, and protect your health.

If you or a loved one has been diagnosed with cancer, there will be a lot on your mind. There's a high degree of uncertainty, as well as the constant fear of change. It is well-known that individuals who have been diagnosed with cancer tend to exhibit distressing feelings. For some, this creates feelings of depression and anxiety. This is totally normal!

When individuals who are suffering from cancer adopt a mindfulness approach, they're able to live in the present moment. They begin to understand that not everything needs to be known and that they should focus on what is currently happening. This allows patients to focus on WHAT they can do, instead of WHY these issues are happening to them.

When you focus your energy on present time, you begin to make significant changes in terms of your lifestyle and mindset. This helps you focus on what you do can to improve your situation, instead of dwelling on what you could have done differently.

Self-Awareness

With mindfulness, you need self-awareness. No matter what the topic is, being self-aware is critical throughout life. When someone is diagnosed with cancer, it's vital that they do not enter a damaging state of denial. Not recognizing that you have cancer for weeks or months could greatly impair your treatment or ability to properly cope in the future.

You will need to make important decisions, which is why you need to be aware of how you're feeling and what's going on. When you practice self-awareness, you begin to understand what your strengths and limitations are. This is so important! To tap into your true self, is a highly rewarding experience. Based on this experience, self-awareness can be an essential part of your healing process.

While focusing on cancer prevention, it is important to be aware of your body and any possible changes that occur. Denying the fact that you've had strange symptoms for three weeks is not a beneficial approach. Being fully aware of your body is a great way to recognize when something might not be right. For many forms of cancer, early intervention significantly increases your risk of survival.

A classic example of being self-aware in terms of cancer is being *breast self-aware*. Knowing YOUR breasts helps you be self-aware of what's abnormal. In fact, the majority of women who experience breast cancer actually identify symptoms on their own. Breast cancer is a prime example, because catching it early can increase your risk of a full recovery.

It's so easy to suppress little red flags that pop up and alert us to something being off in our body. Suppress and deny and maybe it will go away, right? Wrong. This is our body letting us know that something is off. Being self-aware could save your life.

So, if this was me, 20-some years ago, with my cancer diagnosis in one hand and this book in another, I'd be screaming, "so what do I do, lady?!?" But then again, I had just learned how to express anger. ;)

elissa goodman

Here are some ideas about what you can do.

Work with a Coach

Although your high school basketball or track days might be over, that doesn't mean you won't benefit from a coach. Simply put, a life coach is someone who will guide, teach, and encourage you. When you become ill, someone supporting and educating you along your journey is highly beneficial. A cancer coach can help you work through your feelings and overwhelming emotions. The coach will provide you with the education and support you need, in order to not only focus on healing physically, but emotionally and spiritually as well.

It's not uncommon to experience racing thoughts and overwhelming fears. Your coach is someone who can provide you with clarity in times of need. By helping you reduce stress, you can focus on treating your cancer, while increasing your overall quality of life. Some days you might feel like quitting, as you become exhausted both mentally and physically. A coach can motivate you; help you see what you're fighting for. This can ignite your efforts, as you feel empowered, regaining a sense of control.

It's also a really incredible thing to have someone who is invested in you, but not in your immediate family or friend group supporting you. I know when I was diagnosed with cancer, some days I felt like nothing in my world was going right. Everything Marc said was wrong, everything my friends said was inconsiderate. Sometimes you need a neutral third party to come in and tell you it's okay for you to really believe it.

You CAN take control of your health and destiny, which is why a holistic cancer coach can do wonders. You can share your goals and priorities with your coach, so that he or she can focus on what it is you need. Depending on the treatment you choose, your coach can help you adjust and support that treatment method. They will help you make necessary changes to your lifestyle and diet, as this will benefit anyone, regardless of the chosen treatment.

elissa goodman

Perhaps you already have a therapist. He or she can work in this way for you as well. It's important to find someone who is a neutral third party who can really listen to you and go through this journey with you without having any of their own emotions in the situation.

Harness the Benefits of Yoga

When I was going through cancer treatment, I discovered yoga and it saved me. It was a savior for my stress and anxiety. I felt totally bombarded with frightening information, invasive procedures, and had to endure cold clinics and scared stares from the people I loved most. Yoga forced me to clear my mind of the scary stuff and make way for the calming stuff.

If you are currently undergoing treatment, you know how exhausting it can be. Battling with cancer is no easy task, which is why you need to maintain and strengthen your body. When you are physically stronger, you can cope better. There are side effects associated with cancer and cancer treatment, which is why you need to maintain your strength. In turn, this helps you cope better on a mental level. The physical benefits are many, as yoga improves circulation and flexibility, as well as muscle and joint strength.

One of the most beneficial systems that are targeted in yoga is the lymphatic system. This helps individuals with cancer further encourage detoxification. Since deep breathing plays an important role, tired cells gain much-needed oxygen and nutrients.

All of this is great, but there is more, much more! In terms of your psychological wellbeing, yoga does wonders. If you are feeling anxious or tense regarding your condition, yoga will help you achieve a greater sense of self and wellbeing. As we discussed, stress hinders your immune system. Any opportunity you have to reduce stress is highly recommended.

Although regular exercise is highly beneficial, most individuals undergoing cancer treatment simply do not feel like going to the gym or for a morning jog. Yoga however, is a low-impact exercise,

elissa goodman

which targets your whole body. This allows individuals with cancer to regularly exercise, strengthening their body's natural ability to defend itself.

My yoga practice helped get rid of my feelings of depression and extreme anxiety and feel more positive, peaceful, and calm. I felt relief every time I stepped onto that mat. Still to this day, even putting on yoga pants calms me. Yoga is still a part of my life and the benefits are still so important to me. Yoga forces you to breathe deeper and release. Whatever you are worried about when you start your practice, I guarantee it will become less important by the time you're done.

Eat Antidepressant and Anti-Inflammatory Foods

And you thought you were going to get away with not talking about food this chapter! Unfortunately, the foods that you consume not only affect your physical health, but your mental health as well. Depression and anxiety are not uncommon disorders, which are often treated with prescription antidepressants. These often create numerous side effects; and only mask the symptoms, without treating the root cause.

Before you turn to antidepressants, it's important to explore dietary options. There are many foods that promote hormonal and neurochemical balancing. Foods that help synthesize serotonin can significantly improve your mood and emotional wellbeing. Some of the best serotonin-boosting foods include dark leafy greens, turkey, beans, pumpkin seeds, spirulina, sesame seeds, mushrooms, watercress, and legumes.

There are also many foods that increase inflammation in your body and can increase depression or anxiety issues. These include anything processed, sugar, dairy, and gluten. Although you might believe that serotonin is solely located in the brain, 95 percent of your body's serotonin is actually found in your gut.

Your gut health needs support, so that it can release these "feel-good" chemicals. When you consume a poor diet, which is low in nutrients, it is easy for an imbalance to occur. Since your mental health directly influences your physical health, you need to consume a diet that supports healthy brain and gut functioning. Your entire body is connected, so if you load it with junk, you'll feel crappy—physically, mentally, and emotionally. Just like you can't only eat kale and ignore your emotions, you can't only do yoga and eat pizza every night.

Reflexology

If you're not familiar with reflexology, you're not a client of mine. I have been known to send my clients directly from my office to get a reflexology massage. We are blessed in Los Angeles with inexpensive and incredible walk-in reflexology massage places on every other corner. Have you ever discovered something so incredible that you cannot wait to meet someone who does not know about it because you know that sharing your secret will change his or her life? That's how I feel about reflexology.

Reflexology is the application of pressure to various points on your hands, feet, or ears. It is the belief that these specific points correspond to other areas of the body, influencing different systems and organs. When pressed, these areas benefit in terms of functionality.

Reflexologists utilize maps, which have been recognized by practitioners around the world. Your left foot, for example, will correspond to the left side of your body, including all of the valves and organs within that left side. The same is true for your right foot. Since your liver is located on the right side of your body for instance, its reflex area is specifically found on your right foot. Although this practice is not a cure, it is part of an effective, holistic strategy.

Reflexology has the ability to relax individuals, as they cope with feelings of stress. This directly impacts feelings of anxiety, which should be addressed and not bottled up. In turn, this can also help minimize pain and improve mood.

If you're prone to suppressing your emotions, you need to release that tension. Reflexology has been shown to restore balance within the body, as tension is reduced. In fact, many individuals often describe their reflexology experience as total relaxation, increasing energy levels. Fatigue is often associated with cancer treatment, which will, of course, be worsened by suppressed emotions.

Not only are symptoms of stress reduced, but also it's believed that applying pressure to specific areas helps aid in blocked pathways. When energy flow is improved, you're able to promote positive health; and since circulation tends to improve, reflexology can help restore bodily functions.

If you think this is some kind of hoax, I urge you to try it once and I guarantee you'll be hooked. When everything in my life feels like it's about to explode, I go get a reflexology massage. My kids, my fiancé, and my assistant will all attest to the miracle even a 30-minute massage can work on me.

It's important to treat yourself to things that reduce stress, especially while you are battling cancer. If in less than the time it will take you to make dinner you can have all your fears and worries melted away—why wouldn't you?

Keep a Journal

My diagnosis opened the floodgates for my emotions but it was up to me to start processing them. I journaled a bit, but I wish as part of that process that I had written down everything. I wish I had written out the things that pissed me off or made me sad or made me anxious over and over again until they were nothing but words.

Just as art and music therapy have provided benefits to many, journal writing is a hugely beneficial outlet. When you physically write down your thoughts and experiences, you automatically become more self-aware. This is not a new concept, however, as researchers have recognized the benefits of writing for years.

Although journaling most certainly benefits one's emotional wellbeing, it also helps individuals feel better physically. It's a way for you to personally express yourself, without judgment or fear. When you are overwhelmed with emotion, write it down. Not only is this an outlet for your feelings, but also you can go back and reflect. Sometimes we feel emotions but we don't know what to write.

I would recommend getting into the habit of writing for 15–30 minutes every day. Set a timer if needed and even if you are writing out "I have nothing to say" over and over, keep writing it. It's incredibly healing to allow yourself to release and write but also to document your journey. On the days when it feels as though you've made no progress, you have written proof that you have.

This is for you and no one else. It's a place where you feel safe, as you describe your journey. It can be tough to express your feelings and fears, especially to loved ones. You might not want to worry them, or you don't know how to properly express yourself to them. Basically, a journal is one extra step toward releasing stress and built-up negative emotions.

If you don't know what to write about, here are a few suggestions. Remember, this is YOUR personal healing journey, so feel free to write about anything you desire:

- Lists are a great way to really let it all out. You can write a list of your top 20 strengths, a list that displays 50 ways you could positively impact your life, 10 ways your life has changed since your diagnosis, 5 things you are grateful for that day, or whatever else you can think of.

- Letters can help us resolve past conflicts or harbored feelings in which we'd like to let go. Cancer is a major life transition, which will have you thinking about people who have affected your life. If it is someone from your past, then this is a great way to let go of damaging resentment. You can

elissa goodman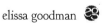

move forward, as you learn to live in the present moment. You can also write letters to those who are currently in your life and mean the world to you. If there are feelings that you haven't expressed to these individuals, you can write letters that they might or might not see. This is for you, as you address your feelings and finish any old business that's hindering your ability to move forward.

- Reflecting on memories or thoughts can help you get your creative juices flowing. When you can't think of anything to write about, choose a phrase or a memory and reflect on it. What does it mean to you? What can you learn from it?

Not everything in your journal needs to reflect your illness or treatment. It's important to stop and count your blessings as well. Perhaps you saw the most magnificent sunrise this morning, which instantly boosted your mood. Write about this experience, as you reflect on the positive aspects of your life.

If you are helping a loved one through his or her cancer journey, it's just as important for you to journal as it is for them. You are feeling huge emotions as well, don't allow yourself to believe that their emotions are the only ones that need to be given attention. Marc didn't repress his emotions at all; he let them out a million times over. We were opposites that way.

He was really angry and I didn't know how to handle it. It scared me because I always thought it was directed at me even though deep down I knew it wasn't. I already felt handcuffed by my emotions that he was sick and taking on his emotions too could've been terrible for both of us. I journaled a lot during his illness and it kept me sane, and relaxed and ready and able to handle the emotions that his emotional response drew up in me.

Marc and I are perfect examples of two ends of the spectrum. He overexpressed everything and I suppressed everything. I'm trying to do everything differently with my girls. I want to make sure they express all their emotions in a contained and healthy way. My oldest daughter is a lot like Marc and my youngest is a lot like me. This is not always easy for me.

It's way easier to fall back into my old patterns. It's easy for me to suppress the fears and anxieties I have about them, but I've worked really hard to make things different for them. I have seen firsthand how emotional turmoil can lead to physical and/or mental illness. When my girls journal, I know that even though they aren't expressing directly to me, they are expressing in some way.

I talk a lot about emotional health with them and try to create an environment in which they feel comfortable opening up. Emotional health means trusting yourself enough to feel what you really want to feel and having the resources to express that in a controlled and safe way.

While you're at the store grabbing your vegetables, grab a journal as well. I've never had a client tell me that taking care of their emotions has hurt them. Beneath what is scary and tumultuous is peace. Let's find it.

"I am safe. I trust my body to release what no longer serves me.
I am divinely guided."

HACK 8:
Disconnection from Self

Did you know that practicing mindfulness could make you more aware of yourself and your surroundings? In fact, our mind can process 126 pieces of information a second. That is a lot of information you're missing out on!

—*Psychology Today*, June 2013

Did you know that a lack of self-awareness is related to both personality and emotional variables?

—Synapse.org

Did you know that grateful people experience less aches and pains?

—Forbes, November 2014

Throughout this book, we have focused a lot on changing our behaviors and habits. Often times, it is easier to take on new things and create new habits than it is to look within and find out why we had our original habits to begin with. Although we are constantly connected with the world around us, we have become more and more disconnected from our true selves.

When we reconnect with ourselves and allow our mind and body to work together, amazing things can happen. How and what you think will affect how you physically feel just as how you feel will affect the way you think. Stress can affect you physically and this physical condition can directly influence your feelings and thoughts. When you are battling cancer or any disease, you might become anxious, stressed, or depressed. It is easy to feel overwhelmed and when your body feels crappy, often times your mind does too. This can influence the way you cope as well as your approach and response to treatment.

Our world is full of constant distractions. In this chaos, it is easy to lose focus. We are disconnected from ourselves, which tends to be the root cause of many problems. If we are not connected to ourselves—how can we be whole? How can our body function at its optimal level if its moving parts are not all on the same page?

Seeking emotional wellbeing is just as important as everything else we have talked about in this book. I think my disconnection from my self was one of the main reasons I got cancer. My diet was crappy, I never made time to work out or allow for downtime, and I was far from being in touch with my emotions. But more important, in the back of my mind, I was always someone who was sick and needy and relied on other people for things. No matter the success I found at work or in relationships, I still felt like I was not good enough and that I did not deserve to take care of myself. I had been carrying around these feelings for a really long time.

When I was 18 years old, my mom took me to see a woman who did horoscope readings. My mom did not like my boyfriend at the time, and, honestly, I think she was hoping this woman would tell me that he was bad news. Instead, the woman told me I would have a serious disease by the time I turned 40 and there was a good chance I would not survive. I did not think that people who had a gift to see into the future were supposed to tell you negative and potentially devastating things like this. You might be able to imagine how jarring that was to hear.

I carried that reading in my body like a death sentence. Every year, I felt like I was looking over my shoulder to see when it would strike. Death was coming for me and I knew it. It all made sense. That is what my weak, useless body was meant to do—to die. I felt broken, but I tucked it inside. It was a big pot of simmering disease and it was coming for me any minute.

When I got diagnosed at 32, the first thing I felt was relief. My horoscope death sentence was scary in its vagueness. Getting this diagnosis gave me details and specifics. My mysterious illness was here. At the time, I thought, "I cannot believe that woman was right." Now, when I look back I think, "I cannot believe I believed her." Listening to her and taking her word as truth was the worst thing I could have ever done.

In so many ways, I am grateful for my cancer. It taught me to slow down, look within, and create a happier and healthier existence for me. With that said, focusing on that toxic prediction probably brought me cancer. Every day I told my body, "I'm waiting for disease." And finally my body said, "Okay, fine, we will give it to you." I was allowing myself to think of someone who deserved or was owed illness. Of course I got sick! I was literally asking for it.

Pain, trauma, and emotional imbalance disconnect us from ourselves. We do not want to feel those things so we figure out how to hide them away. I did not want to face the fear that came with what the horoscope woman told me that day. I tried to sweep it under the rug and, at the same time, I took on the burdens of not having those emotions addressed.

Burdens are far heavier than the events that inspire them. I could have left that appointment and told someone what she said and that it scared me. I could have talked it out and questioned mortality and I might have been able to move on from it. I could have had a conversation with my mom about how it made me feel that she took me there and why the woman would say such a horrible thing and I might have found relief. Instead, I shackled myself to it and carried it around for years allowing it to grow bigger and stronger until it truly overtook me.

I did not think I had the strength or willpower to address the anxieties I had in my life. When they were bad, I placed as many bandages as possible over them until the symptoms died down and I could continue with my life. I was not really living; I was just trying to survive. When my problems became unmanageable, I would finally deal with my problems.

Managing our issues is not anywhere near as important as handling them. We should not be okay with popping a Xanax every time we have a panic attack and then getting through that day and then ignoring it until it comes up again.

It is incredibly important to get to a place where negativity, anxiety, and depression are not ruling your life. Being in that place makes it near impossible to make the changes you need to make for your health and mental wellbeing. We need to learn how to not be afraid of those feelings, how to face them head-on. If you embrace the uncomfortable, that is when BIG shifts start to happen for the better.

The steps to reconnection are not extreme and they are not hard. But they thrive on consistency and dedication. They are a part of a greater but more subtle journey. You will not see results overnight, but one day you will look back and think, "I am so much happier and more at peace now."

Here are my steps to strengthening your wellbeing and reconnecting with yourself:

Have a Practice Every Day

As I mentioned above, consistency is crucial. It is important that you do something every single day that benefits you. It is a reminder that no matter what life throws at you, you can still be in control of how you feel and how you spend your day. Whether it is—yoga, meditation, walking, or hiking—find something that benefits your health and that you can do every day. These practices help you connect physically, mentally, and spiritually, allowing your *whole* self to benefit. You cannot control your manager's mood or the traffic or your doctor's diagnosis, but you can do something for yourself today.

If you do not currently have a daily practice, there is no need to make things complicated. When starting out, create a simple, yet beneficial practice. Start by doing 10 minutes of yoga in the morning. Ten minutes—that is all. If you like it, start doing 20 minutes. Maybe after a few weeks, you want to do 20 minutes of yoga and 15 minutes of meditation every morning.

Starting small and building a practice is a lot more realistic than trying to immediately jump into a huge lifestyle change. Think of a skill you have learned in the past. Chances are, you perfected it by practice—a little bit, slowly until you got it. A daily practice is no different. IF you practice yoga every day for 15 minutes, it will be more beneficial than practicing yoga once a month for two hours.

Each day you will become more in tune with your body. The first day or the first week, maybe even the first month, it won't feel like a huge change. But your mindset will change and you'll feel more aware of the way you feel and how your practice makes you feel.

Writing in a journal is another great beneficial daily practice and can help you track how these feelings change and grow. How you feel on day one will highly differ from how you feel on day twenty. Keeping a journal will remind you of the progress made.

Whatever you choose to do—make it a priority and do not let it fall by the wayside.

Begin Each Day with Gratitude and Affirmations

This is one of the simplest things we can do and yet one of the most effective. In our hectic lives, it is easy to lose sight of the positivity around us. When you have cancer, feeling grateful feels like a lot of work. It is challenging to not focus on the scary, bad stuff and focus on the good. Cancer mounts your life and it feels like it is in charge. How can you be happy about something as small as finding a good parking spot at Whole Foods when you are still a person with cancer? I get that, I really do. And it is not easy to start looking for something good when it feels as though everything is going wrong. But I promise that if you commit to do this for even one week, you will see a difference.

Every day, write down five things that are you are grateful for. Maybe you are grateful for your family, your healthy children, or the roof over your head. Maybe you are grateful that the sun is shining or that your green tea tastes particularly good. Maybe you're grateful that your husband didn't snore last night or that your favorite towel is clean. The point is not to be moving mountains; the point is to be recognizing the good. It is so easy to ignore these gifts or to take them for granted. It is easy to not focus on the little, good stuff and only focus on the big, bad stuff. But these small instances can bring great pleasure.

When you start the day thinking about what you are grateful for, you have already started on a positive note. You are stepping into the day with gratitude, pleasure, and hope. You are telling yourself that some things are shitty, but some things are good and that is a world that is a million times better than 100 percent shitty.

On top of a gratitude journal, starting your day with a positive affirmation is another easy dose of positivity. The simplest one is "all is well." You can say it to yourself a few times in the mirror. "All is well, all is well, all is well." You can also say other affirmations, such as, "I am healthy" or "I am calm" or "I have the power to positively influence my life." Whatever it is, say it a few times and really mean it. Remember, your mind can have positive effects on your health. You need to tell your mind that everything is okay, that *all is well*. Keep repeating it.

Value Yourself

If we were asked if we value ourselves, our answers would be all over the spectrum. But the truth is, most of us do not value ourselves. We do not give ourselves enough time or credit to take care of ourselves. This is saying to yourself that you aren't worth it and decreases your inner value. The way in which you view yourself affects your mental health *and* physical health. Poor self-esteem is not uncommon. We all have some area of our lives that we feel self-conscious about. But if you think healthy, you will naturally achieve more positive health. When you truly value yourself, you will make choices that benefit your wellbeing.

If you or someone you love is currently struggling with cancer, I know the feelings that come with it. It is easy to feel self-hate and feel as though you did something to deserve this. Eliminating negative thoughts and emotions is easier said than done. But a positive mindset can do wonders for you and your health. If you do not value yourself, how can you implement positive change? Your self-perception plays a major role in the way you behave, even if you are not consciously aware.

As humans, we love to compare ourselves to others. In these days, where social media rules the world, it is easy to look at other people's lives and wonder why we cannot have what others have. We spend so much time focusing on other people's strengths that all we can see is our weaknesses.

You are unique and you are special. Being you means that you are someone with your own personal skills, talents, and ideas. When you open yourself up and harness this concept, you open yourself up to possibility. You need to allow yourself to grow into yourself and love yourself. As someone who battled cancer, I know how important it is to believe in your abilities. The way in which you view yourself, and, more important, the things you believe you can achieve, will significantly impact your life.

elissa goodman

Your gratitude journal will help you feel more value in your life but another great exercise is to take a few 10-minute breaks during the day. Do something just for yourself, even if it is just sitting quietly and having a cup of your favorite tea. This will allow you to feel more energetic, relaxed, and creative. It allows you to step back and focus on how you are feeling.

It is empowering to allow yourself to take time for yourself. If you do not feel amazing, do not wallow in it. Step back and ask yourself what you can do to change that. You deserve that. Remind yourself that you have value and things to offer and your happiness matters. Because it does!

Trust Your Gut

I'm not done talking about your gut. We all have an innate superpower and it is called intuition. Your gut knows what is best for you. When you get that feeling in your gut, it is telling you to pay attention. So listen up!

Our innate instincts help us make decisions where the right answer is not obvious. It plays a huge role in the decisions we make. The tricky part is that we are capable of highly complex thoughts and these thoughts make it easy to talk us out of our gut feelings.

When it comes to cancer, choosing your treatment plan is important. You need to trust your gut when it comes to the people you work with and the plans you make. If you meet someone and something feels slightly off, that is your gut telling you to stay away. Listen to it!

Now, as a caveat, there are many factors to everything, so a gut feeling doesn't have to be the sole decider in the choices you make. Sometimes fear can be mistaken for a gut feeling. Pay attention, use logic, and see how your gut feelings change.

The same is true for cancer prevention. If you feel as though something does not feel right with your health, what should you do? You got it, listen to your gut! There is no harm in getting things checked out. Best case, you ate something a little funky and it will pass in a couple days. Worst case, there is something more serious developing.

When it comes to cancer, the earlier you catch it, the better. So often we ignore red flags because we don't want the worst-case scenario to be true. But the sooner you rule that out, the better. And if it is the worst-case scenario, it is only getting worse the longer you wait. The earlier you are, in terms of cancer development, the more options you will have. You are an expert when it comes to your own body. Do NOT brush off symptoms that are abnormal. Be proactive, trust your gut!

Surround Yourself with Goodness

You know those people who light up any room? Those people who make you feel good, simply by being in their presence? These are the types of people you need to surround yourself with. How you personally feel is easily influenced by those around you.

We are social beings who thrive on being loved and cared for. Think about the connections you have with friends and family members. Why is it that you feel so strongly for them? For the most part, it's because these people bring joy to your life. They encourage and nurture you.

When I went through my cancer experience, I had some incredible people in my life. But I also had some not-so-incredible people. These people were fun to go out with but when the times got tough, they did not know how to be there for me. It was not totally their fault. I allowed them to treat me this way. I thought it was something I was doing, that I was overwhelming them or talking about my cancer too much.

It is not that these are bad people for you to be with; it is just that they might be bad for you right now. You want people who bring positivity into your life. They do not absorb your negativity; they are just being a light to which you can only shine next to. If you are undergoing treatment, this can make a world of difference. Surround yourself with people who help you relax and enjoy yourself. A little bit of laughter can fill a room with hope and change negative emotions into a more positive experience.

Guess what? When you're more positive, you will attract positive people. A few weeks into your gratitude journal, you will start to see this happen. It is amazing how positive people work like magnets; they seem to attract one another. It is your choice who you spend your time with. If there are individuals who bring you down, then you need to consider your options.

Negativity is toxic for anyone's wellbeing. If you have cancer, you need to avoid negativity at all costs. It's always going to seem easier to talk about the bad, but you have to push yourself to focus on the good. Eventually, you will see no other way of living your life!

Take Time to Disconnect

I remember when my dad first got a pager. In case of an emergency, he could be paged and then he had to find a phone and call. At that time, the pager felt like such a huge technological advance that connected us to people so easily and quickly. Well, we have grown a million miles since then. We live in a society that is constantly connected. You do not need me to tell you this. Our cellphones are constantly in our hands—everyone is just a call or text away. Have you ever gotten frustrated because you cannot reach someone for an hour? We are expected to constantly be in communication.

It is important that you take time out of your day to disconnect from all of this. Emails, gossip, and news stories can make it challenging to unwind. When you disconnect, you allow your body to relax, it stops looking for constant stimulation from the outside world. It is easy to spend hours every day checking your email, Facebook, Instagram, Twitter, etc. There is nothing wrong with being connected, but it is as important to know how to disconnect.

What if you spent the time you spent on Facebook taking a walk? What if you turned off that TV show you do not even care about and did a little yoga instead? Eliminating distractions can be a blessing and you will reap the benefits.

Take Some Herbs

There are so many wonderful, natural herbs that are helpful with inducing relaxation and helping you calm down and reduce your anxiety and depression. I'm only naming a few of my favorites, and I always recommend talking to your doctor before taking any supplements.

Ashwagandha

This is one of my favorite adaptogenic herbs. An adaptogen is a botanical that greatly improves your body's ability to adapt to stress. It can help build strength, energy, stamina, endurance, and improve mental clarity.

5-HTP (5-hydroxytryptophan)

This can help your depression by increasing your serotonin, a calming neurotransmitter. DO NOT take with any prescription antidepressant or antianxiety medications.

Kava

This can help relieve panic attacks and reduce overall anxiety. Do not consume alcohol. Ask your doctor first if you are taking other medications.

Gaba

An amino acid, gamma-aminobutyric acid, is responsible for decreasing anxiety in the nervous system, it also helps relax muscles.

You are in charge of you. You are in charge of how you feel. You are in charge of how you think. Cancer won't kill itself. It is a new road you have to be willing to explore. You will need to stay motivated, so do you want someone who is encouraging and kind in your ear or someone who is mean and degrading?

Take care of yourself, give yourself permission to take care of yourself and make your life your priority. It is not always easy to relax and disconnect and take "me" time. But you deserve it. And you need it. So go get it. Every day!

"I give myself permission to flourish in joy."

HACK 9:
Lack of Solid Sleep

Did you know that an estimated 50 to 70 million Americans currently suffer from a sleep disorder that hinders their level of daily productivity, as well as their health and longevity?

—Institute of Medicine (US) Committee on Sleep Medicine and Research, 2006

Did you know there are around 90 sleep disorders affecting us today?

—International Classification of Sleep Disorders, 2001

Did you know that melatonin could help prevent cancer and aid in cancer treatment?

—Dr. Joseph Mercola, Mercola.com, March 2013

Sometimes I think our country has a bit of posttraumatic stress disorder (PTSD). We are so ruined from the years and years of being told that the way to health is through sugar-free Jell-O, hiding from butter, and spending two hours daily at the gym. We became the "just do it" culture—if you wanted something, you have to bust your ass until you get it. I'm all about hard work but there can be a fine line between hard work and punishment. Our bodies cannot survive the beating every day, they need a lot of refueling. Your body needs nourishment, relaxation, and TLC; it needs to be told that you are on its team, that you are in this together.

One area where Americans really got it wrong is sleep. In our culture, sleeping too much is considered a sign of weakness. Sleep is for the sick or lazy college students with no real responsibilities.

elissa goodman

We commend those who survive on just a few hours of sleep a night and apologize for sleeping in.

Growing up, my parents definitely thought this way. They shot out of bed early every morning to work out and to get a head start on their day. They believed you cannot get ahead and be successful if you sleep too much. It was a pressure-filled household with that mentality, because I LOVED to sleep and I definitely needed more sleep than them. When I didn't get my sleep, I got sick every time.

Marc beat to the same drum as my parents, maybe that's why I married him—they do say you marry your parents after all! He always felt there was something else that he could be doing that was better than sleep. He was up every morning at 5 AM to go to a 530 AM Barry's Bootcamp class. In his mind, and in the mind of so many of us, sleeping just got in the way of the things that made him healthy and productive.

Listen, I'm all about working out and using your time wisely to relieve stress from your workload. But what we have gotten so wrong is that sleep is not important. The old idea that if you can survive the day on a few hours of sleep, you are fine is killing us.

I am a sleeper; I always have been. I go to bed around 10 PM and sleep until 7 AM. When I vacation, I sleep even more. I love sleep. When I would watch Marc get out of our bed every morning to go work out, my heart ached. In his mind, working out was the best thing for his health. In my mind, I knew he needed rest.

Lack of solid sleep is a chronic condition that affects most Americans. You probably know about common sleep conditions, such as insomnia or narcolepsy. But there are more than 90 sleep disorders currently affecting Americans. Chances are high you have one. If you wake up in the night to go to the bathroom, if you wake up in the night and check your phone, if you have trouble falling asleep, if you have trouble getting out of bed—these are all symptoms of sleep conditions. Sound familiar?

The short-term effects of bad sleep are not great—it leaves us cloudy, irritable, and much more likely to reach for coffee and sugar. The long-term effects are scary. It increases your chances of diabetes, hypertension, depression, heart attack, obesity, cancer, stroke, and more. It weakens immune function and allows disease to thrive. In fact, when sleep deprived, it's been shown that tumor growth accelerates.

Not getting enough sleep also increases your risk of stress-related disorders as well as leading to heart complications, mood disorders, and stomach ulcers. A well-slept body can regulate insulin levels, repair damages, maintain controlled blood pressure, regulate hormones, and more. A body that has not gotten enough sleep is a ticking time bomb for disease.

If you have a cancer diagnosis, sleep is more important than ever. When you sleep, your body heals. It is common for cancer to hinder your ability to fall or stay asleep. You might have depression or anxiety that prevents you from sleeping. Medications, chemotherapy, and radiotherapy can cause side effects that include interrupting your sleep cycle.

The odds might feel as though they are against you, but it's my goal to get your sleep on track. Sleep is your recovery period, it's where your mind can rest and your body can heal. So the first thing you need to get out of your mind is that you do not need it. You DO need it and you need a lot of it. According to the US National Institutes of Health, nine-and-a-half hours of solid sleep at least seven months out of the year is the *minimum* required to beat cancer, diabetes, heart disease, and depression. If you just said, "I have not slept that much in decades," you are not alone. Most people I know sleep about six hours a night. But sleep is a gift of recovery and so crucial to your healing journey.

When I was diagnosed with cancer, I knew it was my body asking me to slow down. This is often the case. Have you ever noticed that you get sick when you are really busy? It's your body telling you that it needs rest, you have not slept enough, and you are not taking care of yourself. It's often much easier to see in retrospect, but sometimes cancer and disease presents itself to force you to take a break. The best thing you can do is honor your body's wish.

So how can you get more sleep? Read on.

Sleep in a Cool, Dark Room

Most people sleep in the dark, but don't know how significant darkness and light are to our sleep schedules. Up until 1910, when the light bulb became affordable to everyone, our bodies functioned in their most natural state: we slept when it was dark and woke when it was light. During that time people slept 9–10 hours a night. When it begins to get dark, our pineal gland naturally produces a hormone known as melatonin, which helps our bodies prepare for sleep. These days, it's so common for people to take melatonin as a supplement to sleep because their bodies are not producing it naturally. This is a problem!

How much light is in our environment will dictate how much melatonin we produce. When we are exposed to light, signals are sent from our retina to our brain, which then tells our pineal gland to stop releasing melatonin. We also experience a rise in our body temperature and a spike in cortisol. When it's dark outside, our pineal gland is turned on. Melatonin levels rise dramatically, creating reduced alertness and focus. Our body is preparing for sleep.

Ideally, you don't want to experience decreased melatonin levels until dawn. Although our bodies are on a biological clock in terms of our wake-sleep cycle, melatonin will not be produced at night unless you are in a dark or dim setting. And melatonin isn't just important for sleeping, it also protects and supports your immune system, targets inflammation and free-radical damage, working as an effective antioxidant. It also inhibits the growth of cancer cells and triggers the destruction of cancer cells that do develop.

For those undergoing chemotherapy, melatonin has been shown to reduce toxicity. It's especially beneficial to those who suffer from reproductive cancers. Even cancer cells have melatonin receptors, which allow this hormone to latch on and counteract cell growth. Due to melatonin's ability to calm reproductive hormones, it's believed to be especially useful when treating cancers such as breast, ovarian, prostate, testicular, and endometrial.

You need it to heal!

Perhaps this has had you add melatonin to your grocery store shopping list. As much as I love supplements to enhance our health, it's crucial to get the things that your body produces naturally, in the most natural way. Taking melatonin doesn't repair the core issue. You need to create an environment in which your body is creating melatonin itself.

Which means, turn off your overhead lights at 7 or 8 PM. Use lamps and dimmed lighting in the evening. Get out of the habit of doing light-stimulating activities, such as watching TV or being on your phone right before bed. I try to not check my phone after 8 PM. I know, I know. It's a hard habit to break. Most of us are used to looking at our phones last thing before we go to sleep. If you absolutely cannot disconnect, make sure the brightness is all the way down at minimum and try to not look at it at least an hour before you sleep.

If you read before bed—first of all, good for you!—but use lamps instead of harsh overhead lights. Even the common alarm clocks that display the time are emitting enough light to disrupt your melatonin production. Make sure you are looking around your room and seeing complete darkness. Remove any gadgets, phones, computers, or clocks that have light.

If you get up during the night, try not to turn on any lights. This brief moment of light exposure can inhibit or cease melatonin production. Your brain will assume it's time to prepare for the day when you really might still need another four or five hours of sleep!

It's also important that you get time in the sun during the day. This will help your body produce more melatonin at night because the amount of melatonin that's produced is based off the contrast of light during the day to the darkness at night. If you spend all day in a low-lit room, your melatonin production will not be optimized. Try to spend some time outside when you first wake up. Simply sitting outside with your morning tea could be hugely beneficial to your circadian rhythm. The bright light sends a clear message that it's now daytime, which also makes weak light signals less confusing to your brain at night.

When it comes to temperature, our bodies are extremely sensitive. Your bedroom should be ideally between 60 and 68 degrees while sleeping. When you sleep, your body drops to its lowest temperature, typically about four hours after you've fallen asleep. When your room matches this natural drop, your sleep is benefitted. Ever notice how when you take a hot bath before you go to bed, you sleep so much better? That's because when you get out of the bath, your temperature drops, mimicking your body's natural cycle. Signaling your body that it's time to rest allows it time to get prepared to put you to sleep. A cool, dark room is step one!

Get to Bed by 10 PM

Perhaps I subconsciously saved this chapter for the end of my book because I feared losing readers too early on. Perhaps you read "get to bed by 10 PM" and laughed out loud. For many of us, that's a far-off fantasy. I get it. I work a long day and then still want to have plenty of time for family in my evenings. If I go to yoga, sometimes I don't start my nights with my family until 8 PM. And you better believe my teenagers aren't volunteering to go to bed at 10 PM. BUT, hear me out.

It was not until the early 1930s, that we began to understand more about brain activity and what actually occurs when we sleep. Based on electroencephalography (EEG) scans, it was found that our brains are really active during our sleep cycle, not switched off, as was originally believed. As mentioned, our nervous system is highly sensitive to light, which triggers our ability to sleep.

Getting to bed at 10 PM allows you to get maximum restorative sleep. Between the hours of 10 PM and 2 AM is the most beneficial sleeping period, as this is when our natural internal clock slows after the sun goes down. Research has shown that between those hours, one hour of sleep is quality enough to be worth two hours of sleep. Not that you should count that against your nine hours! Going to bed at 10 PM allows your body to be in tune with its natural cycle. Aiming for nine hours of sleep helps your body naturally detoxify, repair, and heal.

It's important to create a routine that you can stick to most days. I know it's tempting to sleep in on the weekends, but the more you create a set cycle, the better quality of sleep you will get. When it comes to bedtime routines, choose activities that will help you sleep and relieve stress. I love deep breathing, aromatherapy, or doing a little meditation before I get into bed. Once my face is washed, my teeth are brushed, and my alarm is set, it allows my body to disconnect completely.

Many of us feel as though 10 PM is not an option, but if we just decide to do it, it's not that difficult. Try to make sleeping and a bedtime routine a priority. You'll immediately feel the difference.

Take an Afternoon Nap

Somewhere in the time when we started shaming ourselves for sleeping too much, we got rid of naps for anyone over the age of five. What a shame! Many cultures celebrate and encourage daytime napping and I completely agree. In Europe, many offices close for an hour in the afternoon solely so it's employees can take an afternoon nap.

Although we might view napping as a lazy activity, it actually helps boost the immune system, relieve tension, and help reverse some of the negative effects associated with a bad night's rest.

Again, environment is important. Try to find a cool, dark place and utilize earplugs and an eye mask, if needed. Nap for no longer than 30 minutes so you don't incite any feelings of grogginess.

Often times, when our to-do list piles up and the day doesn't seem to have enough hours, we feel like we don't even have time to stop for a coffee, let alone take a nap. Truth is, giving yourself 30 minutes to decompress and take a nap will actually revitalize your energy and help you sleep better that evening. Win-win!

Go Tech-Free

I mentioned earlier the importance of turning off your phone, but I know that's a really hard one to tackle, so I want to really stress the importance of turning off your devices.

Individuals of all age (especially the younger generations) are going to bed with their smartphone as close to them as possible. Amazingly, 95 percent of individuals between the ages of 18–29 years old are going to bed with their phone next to them. A quarter of these individuals do not silence their phone, meaning that their sleep can be disrupted by incoming calls and texts. Although the noise and possible light from your phone can affect your sleep, it doesn't stop there. Our cell phones emit electromagnetic radiation. This directly affects our ability to sleep and repair our body.

As technology continually develops, our society needs to adapt. However, there are certain aspects of technology that do not agree with our natural physiology. Your bedroom is supposed to be a place of rest and tranquility, so treat it that way. One of the other biggest concerns is having a television in the bedroom.

You might be someone who enjoys background noise while you sleep, but the continuous glow of your television set will most certainly impact your melatonin levels. For many younger individuals, where there's a television, there's often a gaming system. If you're someone who plays video games in your room before bed, this can actually cause an increase in cortisol levels and affect your ability to sleep.

I know it's not easy. I know many of us use our phones as alarms or want to be able to be reached in case of an emergency. On the iPhone, there's the option to put your phone on "Do Not Disturb" or you can "Allow Calls From" your favorites list or specific groups that you indicate. You can also mark to receive "Repeated Calls" from someone who calls you a second time within three minutes. And no one expects you to be up at 4 AM to get that email that came in from London. Allowing yourself to relax is crucial. You have options to cover all your bases; don't let technology be the reason you aren't healing.

Outside of food, sleep is one of the areas in my field that I've spent a lot of time researching. I could not resist giving you a few other of my favorite sleep tips:

- When the days get shorter in fall and winter, we need more sleep—let your body cooperate with the natural light and dark cycles of the day and allot at least an extra hour of sleep during those months.

- I don't promote an all-raw diet for many reasons, but notably because I believe our bodies need a calming, grounding hot meal with some gluten-free carbs at night in order to settle our energy so we can sleep. An all-raw diet can actually provide too much energy to your body and, yes, that can be a bad thing.

- If you tend to wake up in the middle of the night, specifically between 1–3 AM, you should eat a little protein with fat before bed. Try a warm homemade almond milk or a handful of pumpkin seeds.

- Stress will keep you up! It brings up cortisol, which keeps you awake. Try a reflexology foot massage, an infrared sweat session, a leisurely walk for 20 minutes each day,

 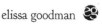

yoga, or lay on your back with your feet elevated over your heart for 15 minutes.

- Get your blood work done if you are having trouble sleeping. This can alert you to any chronic infection that might be affecting your sleep. These are stressful on the body and can affect your adrenal health. If you have a chronic infection, your diet can be instrumental in helping you regain your health.

If all of your efforts are not impacting your ability to sleep, there is one supplement combination I love. It's called Dr. Whitaker Restful Night Essentials, you can take it alone or pair it with magnesium. When Marc passed away, it felt like it was a struggle to get me and my girls a good sleep. I knew how important it was while we were grieving, but, of course, we were all having trouble. Grief is overpowering and can combat any habits we have created. Dr. Whitaker provided a natural way for us to get the sleep we needed. It's the only product I recommend to my clients.

I feel passionately about sleep. To me, it's like wearing a seat belt. It's easy, simple, and can save your life. Why wouldn't you do it? We need sleep to heal. We need it to properly function and to make smart choices throughout the day. If you have made it this far with my book, you are committed to your health. You want to heal and you want to get rid of that cancer and live your best life. I know you do.

Sleeping is such a huge part of this process. Give yourself permission to demand that you get this. It's so easy to let other things get in the way, or let outside sources convince us that going to bed at 10 PM is insane. Maybe your husband is dying to watch one more episode of *Game of Thrones*, or your daughter wants to do some late night online shopping. Perhaps there is laundry to be done or you want to work on your novel in bed. Maybe you do not want to be rude when your friend suggest dinner at 8:30 PM. You probably feel like you do not have the ability to get in bed at 10 PM. You do.

Years ago, I never thought that was a possibility. Once I made it a habit, it seems crazy that I would do anything else. I learned many lessons through my individual journey with cancer, but the biggest one was how crucial it is to slow down. Marc felt like if he stopped moving, he'd stop forever. I felt as though my body was begging me to stop moving. In his mind, working out and staying on top of work made him feel in control of his life and his health. Nothing could stop him.

The thing is, something was trying just to slow him, not stop him. He had not taken a break since I knew him. He was always going, never disconnected, constantly working and moving. He was so full of life—and loved and adored by so many for that. But at the end of the day, he did not know how to release that and give himself some relief.

When I was sick, I felt like such a baby. I wanted to sleep in, relax, and cut back at work. At the time, I felt a bit like failure. I did not have the stamina or motivation to power up when my body was begging me to power down. I am so grateful that I listened to the voice that told me to relax.

We feel like we are succumbing to illness, we want to put up a fight. But fighting cancer is not about how busy and active you can be. It's not about maintaining your exact same life. It's about making an environment in which the cancer cannot thrive. When you take good care of yourself and get good sleep, the cancer starts to suffocate. Chances are it's going to pack its bags and leave.

Release any idea you have that nine hours of sleep is a luxury. It's a necessity, like water. Don't feel shamed into thinking that if you are getting that much sleep you are not doing enough. You are in charge of your life and you are in charge of what you demand of it. If you want to go to bed, go. I highly recommend it.

"I thank my body for restoring and renewing while I sleep."

elissa goodman

HACK 10:
Build Your Cancer-Fighting Environment

The minute you get diagnosed with cancer, the opinions start flying in. Your neighbor's sister had cancer. Your daughter's best friend's mom's cousin had cancer. Your babysitter knows a guy on the west side who cures cancer with his hands.

It's an overwhelming moment: whom do you trust?

When it feels like a life-or-death moment, do you try everything?

One of your choices is to do what Marc did. He trusted his doctors and followed their treatment plan to the letter. He put his fate in his doctors' hands. They called all the shots and he didn't question any of their decisions or recommendations. In hindsight, I can tell you, that was the worst mistake of our lives.

I am not here to bash doctors. They are smart, capable, well-trained human beings who do a lot of good. They have a lot of answers, and they often know how to ask the right questions. With that said, no one, not the highest-ranking doctor in the world, knows you like you do.

Cancer is not like getting a cold or strep throat. There's not one obvious cause or one obvious solution. Oncologists are surely doing their best to tackle cancer as they know best, but at the end of the day, unless they can act as your therapist, nutritionist, emotional support, gym coach, and friend, they cannot give you all the answers regarding your unique cancer case. Oncologists have spent years and years in school studying drugs. They know how to prescribe you drugs, but guess what? Drugs are not the only answer and they often times can be a part of the problem.

But, you have a choice. You have the choice to become smarter than the oncologist and take your health into your own hands. You have the choice to question what you're told, do your own research, and build your own cancer-fighting team.

You have the choice to seek out alternative treatment or to combine alternative treatments with the oncologist's recommendations. You have the choice to make educated and instinctual moves that are right for you and your body. Remember these words: *trust your gut!*

Step One: Finding the Right Doctor Support

The first oncologist I went to see was highly recommended and was considered to be at the top of his field. I immediately felt turned off by him. His space was sterile and unwelcoming, his energy was cold and indifferent. He was arrogant and definitely had a god complex. I was scared out of my mind and, in a lot of ways, liked the comfort of being told what to do. He took charge and we immediately started preliminary testing.

Every time I had to go back to him to get my test results, I dreaded it. It was extremely depressing. It was clear I was just another cancer case to him and that he had no genuine interest in me. In fact, he never called me by my name. During this time, everyone in my life was really scared and freaked out. My family and loved ones wanted answers and they wanted to hear that I was going to be okay.

I wanted to be able to go to him and get the answers and the support in this new and scary situation but he couldn't provide any of that. He made me feel way worse than I already felt. He told me there was no one better than him and that going to another doctor would be a waste of my time.

Always the rebellious type, I took my results to a second doctor to see if I could make progress elsewhere. This doctor had a similar disposition to the first doctor and I started thinking that this was just the way it was going to be and I just had to get used to it.

During this time, my mom was at a conference in Europe and heard a radiation oncologist speak. She approached him after his speech and told him about my diagnosis. In an insane coincidence, he happened to practice at Saint John's Hospital in Santa Monica. I went to see him when he returned and it was a magical moment. His office was comfortable and inviting, somehow he had made a beautiful oasis in a big, cold hospital. He was funny and open and honest and warm. He asked me about life, he asked me about my stress levels. He told me I needed to deal with my emotions, focus on a healthier diet, and get better exercise. At the time, I was doing hardcore exercise, he suggested I try yoga to keep me calm and get me back in touch with my body. I felt safe with him; I felt like I could be honest about how I was feeling and what I was going through. I finally felt like I found my home and someone who truly cared.

You should never be afraid to explore all your options. If I hadn't followed my gut instinct, things could have turned out very different for me.

The first oncologist wanted me to do a full blast of radiation and chemotherapy and to freeze my eggs. The second oncologist wanted me to do a full blast of chemotherapy. The third oncologist wanted me to do localized radiation and suggested I start being more honest and vocal about the emotional turmoil I was going through and how I could start making healthier choices in my life.

Sometimes the last thing you want to do is keep trekking from doctor's office to doctor's office. I get that. But I promise you that finding the right doctor is always worth the pursuit.

elissa goodman

Here is how I knew the third oncologist was the right choice for me:

- He listened to me and respected my opinion.
- He allowed me to ask as many questions as I wanted and gave me plenty of time to feel comfortable with what was happening. He even gave me his direct line so I could call if I had questions or concerns outside of his regular work hours.
- He asked questions about my overall life: Was I happy? Was I stressed? How bad was my anxiety? Had I experienced any trauma in my life? Was my childhood nurturing and supportive? What was my health like as a kid? And most important, he showed true interest in my answers.
- He was open to helping me with alternative lifestyle approaches during my treatment.

Here is my advice for finding the right doctor.

- Buy a journal and take it with you to every appointment. Take notes and record how you're feeling. This also helps ensure you don't miss any information and feel overwhelmed when you leave.
- Bring a family member or friend. Don't try to go through this alone. Some days can be overwhelming and it's important to have a second pair of eyes and ears. It also helps to have someone there who might have questions you don't think of in the moment.
- Record the session on your phone. Nowadays, that's easy! This will allow you to review and absorb the information and/or replay it for loved ones who couldn't make the appointment with you.
- Be honest about seeking a second and/or third opinion. A good doctor with your best interests in mind will understand your need to seek other opinions and might even be able to recommend a reputable doctor for you to get in touch with.

- If you have friends or family members who have any information about a great doctor, it's always worth talking to them.

- Know when to accept your diagnosis and take action. Second and third opinions are smart. When two, three, or more doctors who you respect all have corresponding opinions, it's a good time to listen and move forward with a treatment plan.

Step Two: Get Emotional Support

I had found a doctor who made me feel calm and confident and he wanted me to address my emotions, so I was going to. Dealing with my emotions provided a huge learning curve. I was really young and my cancer diagnosis was scary for me and my loved ones. I felt embarrassed and exposed that I had cancer. I felt like an imposition to my family and friends and I wanted to be able to handle it on my own. I didn't feel like I knew how to balance my own inner emotions along with the new emotions coming from the outer world.

Here are the things I think I did right.

- I started meditating to become more aware of my body and be in touch with my feelings. Boy, was this not easy. I couldn't keep my brain calm. But I kept trying, every day. Strangely enough, there would be periods of quiet time when I would get radiation. I would lay on this table alone in a room beforehand and I had to lay still. I relished those quiet times in which my phone wasn't ringing and no one was asking me how I was. In a weird way, I think that was my true time of meditation.

- I wrote down everything I was feeling in a journal to release my stress. It helped to process my fear and anger in a safe environment. Often, I found myself writing the same thing over and over again until one day it didn't bother me as much.

elissa goodman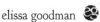

- I found a fabulous therapist who I ended up staying with for thirteen years. He was a lifesaver and together we worked through a lot of the emotional barriers I had put up throughout the years. He forced me to be authentic and called me out if he thought I wasn't telling the whole story or the truth.

- I started doing yoga. It helped me breathe better and calm my mind.

- I walked for at least 20 minutes a day to clear my head and be outside in nature. During this time, I was still working and those breaks felt like solace from my crazy, chaotic life.

- I got massages once a week to help physically release tension and stress.

Here are the things I think I did wrong.

- I talked to too many people about my diagnosis. I was scared and was hoping that if I just told enough people, someone would have a magic solution for me. The way I had dealt with things up until that point in my life was to either sweep it under the rug or find someone else to fix it. When I got my diagnosis, I totally went back into "someone come and save me" mode. Turns out, nobody had a magic solution but a lot of people had an opinion or a story or a fear or a strong feeling about my diagnosis. Their intentions were good, but it became so overwhelming. I couldn't take on their fears *and* my own.

- On top of that, I reveled in being taken care of and showered with love. It sounds a bit creepy and perhaps kind of messed up but there was a part of me that just wanted to soak in all this love. I loved the support I was receiving and being on people's minds, but at some point you have to be mentally committed to feeling better and not wanting to stay in your sickness. I wish I had found a better balance of appreciating the immense and amazing support I received, but also demanding that I got better by learning I could do it for myself and I didn't need all these other people to step up.

- I felt incredibly sorry for myself and at times that it completely paralyzed me. I had a feeling the world was out to get me. I would ask myself, how did that horoscope woman know I was going to have this serious illness when I was 18 years old? I allowed myself to be consumed in a world of shame and blame in moments which my body really needed myself to be focused on how I would heal, not how I got here.

Being Someone Else's Emotional Support System

When Marc was diagnosed, we had already gone through this once, so I felt like I could really support him. Something about his diagnosis seemed scarier than mine, it was more aggressive but the doctors assured us he would live. As you might imagine, it was really hard to provide support to someone who didn't really know how to tell me what he needed. This is such a normal, natural response to someone being in a stressful and scary position in his or her life.

Everyone is different—some people want to be doted on and others want their diagnosis to fade into the woodwork.

Here is what helped with Marc's diagnosis.

- I stayed optimistic for both of us. We had been through this before and I had survived so I was sure he would too.

- I used this as an opportunity to help him look at what wasn't working for him. I supported him and encouraged him to make better choices. I tried to help him make healthier food choices and manage his stress. I tried to get us to bed earlier and show him more nurturing love. I encouraged him to let go of issues that burdened him and deal with emotional baggage. I encouraged him to see his therapist more often.

- One of his friends started a weekly email to keep everyone informed about his progress. Now, there are great websites in which you can post updates as well. This was a game changer for us. It was exhausting answering phone calls and emails and continuing to talk about his condition over and over again.

- I always made sure a friend or family member was at his doctor's appointments with him if I couldn't be there. Before the visit, we wrote down all his questions and concerns to discuss with the doctor and took detailed notes so we had an accurate record of what was said.

When you are vulnerable and in the hospital, it's really cool to have the love, nurture, and support of others. But it can also be overwhelming to always have people asking you about your disease or letting other people bring their own baggage into it. I think it's important to tell people what you need. I wish I could have expressed my expectations at the time. Just having the ability to say, "I love you and I care about you but right now I need some space" or "I need you to call and check on me because it feels awful when you don't, but just know I might not call you back." Nowadays it's so easy to send a text just to remind people you are thinking about them, I think that's really important.

When Marc was in the hospital, there was a young guy in his 30s there who also had Hodgkin's lymphoma. He was a friend of a friend, and he was having a bone marrow transplant (like Marc was) and I would visit him when I visited Marc. It was an isolating place. Visitors had to wear protective clothing and masks. Marc had tons of friends, so someone was there visiting him every day, but this guy had no one visiting him. His family lived out of state and he was all alone. He was going through this bout of illness but was overall healthy and was sure to recover.

One day, I went to visit him and he wasn't there. He had passed. I was so overcome with the feeling that he didn't have the emotional support to carry on. It was heartbreaking to see and I will forever be grateful for all the people who poured out their love and support for Marc. He didn't survive, but every day he had a smiling and caring face coming to see him and that is a beautiful thing.

Here is what didn't help with Marc's diagnosis.

- I have to admit, there is one huge thing I regret in all of this. Marc and I were so carried away with handling our own emotions and we had no clue how to present all this to the girls. They were six and nine at the time and sharing this all with them did not feel right. We tried to hide it from them or sugarcoat details; we were not upfront with them most of the time and I would not advise that for anyone else.

  It's hard to tell them bad news when they are so young, but kids are so instinctual and I think we ended up losing their trust a bit. I wish I had had more guidance about how to deal with that situation. We tried to keep their lives as normal as possible but it was so hard. Marc became extremely sick and we didn't want them to know how bad it was, but I think we did them a disservice.

  When Marc's days were numbered, all his friends and family gathered in his room to say goodbye. I was taking the girls in but they didn't know that this would be the last time they would see him. I was scared and I wanted this to not be real for them. I think looking back I was overcome with denial and I did not have the tools to deal with this and I had not sought them out. The girls came into this alarming room filled with people saying goodbye and I think it really frightened them. It did not give them the chance to prepare and work through some initial emotions so they could make the most of this time with him.

  I have to say, that's my biggest regret in all of this. Every child is different but my advice if you are dealing with something similar would be to get professional support. Do the research and figure out how to take care of your children during this time. It's crucial.

- I learned another big lesson during Marc's cancer fight. He had so many people who wanted to visit him—work people, family, old friends. Some of these people were people he didn't like, but I never knew how to tell them no when they asked if they could visit. He ended up kind of being held hostage by these unwelcome visitors and that is no way to spend your last few months. It became more about pleasing these people, they needed to please themselves and we allowed it to happen.

This is your time; it's not the time to make unwanted reconciliations or to help others feel better about guilt they might be carrying. Give yourself the ability to say no.

Step Three: Understand the Importance of Nutritional Support

Before I got diagnosed, my diet was a rollercoaster. I started my day with a big cup of coffee with Sweet N Low and either a bagel with cream cheese or a muffin. When I felt like I was coming down for that high, I grabbed for sugar—a cookie or a piece of candy. We would get a big ol' deli sandwich for lunch, loaded with processed meats or tuna and mayo. Then dinner usually meant business meetings at a steakhouse where the healthiest thing on my plate was creamed spinach. I truly have no memory of eating salads back then. Even though we were eating so much junk, Marc and I were always interested in the latest and newest craze—what was the fastest way to get thin and look good? It was the era of fad diets and food crazes and there was not one we did not try. It's crazy to me to look back now and think that we didn't see the connection between eating bagels every morning and feeling bloated all day! We were so far from being educated about what was good for us and we listened to every marketing ploy around.

Nutrition being a part of the cancer conversation is a new topic but, in my opinion, it is possibly the most important one. The past few decades in the food world are extremely important in terms of understanding cancer and disease. We have moved so far away from the basics of eating fresh, nutrient-dense foods. We consume zero-calorie desserts and no-fat cheese without even blinking an eye, but this should be a huge red flag for us all.

Diet affects cancer both directly and indirectly. Nutrients directly impact the mechanisms by which cancer cells grow and spread. They indirectly help control the cancer, by changing the surrounding biochemical conditions that either encourage or discourage the progression of malignant disease.

Diets high in unhealthy fats and refined carbohydrates make you more likely to become overweight, which in turn increase your risk of tumor recurrences. Additionally, obese men are at significantly greater risk of developing more aggressive prostate cancer.

Foods that are loaded with trans fats, including margarine, hydrogenated oils, baked goods, and convenience foods, can impair the body's anticancer defenses by depressing the activity of natural killer cells. On the other hand, a diet of healthy fats increases natural killer cells activity. Natural killer cells play a key role in preventing metastasis, which is the process of cancer of spreading.

I don't believe cancer or any other degenerative condition is a disease. I think it's a reaction or symptom. I know my cancer was a reaction to the choices I was making. I wasn't a big smoker and I drank within reason, but I was pounding sugar, coffee, and processed foods, and my emotional stress was out of control. I was continually pushing my feelings inside and not dealing head-on with any of my frustrations, anxieties, sadness, or insecurities.

elissa goodman

Here is what I would do again.

- I changed my diet to include at least 50 percent raw plant-based alkaline foods. Salads and vegetables became the main star of my diet.

- I started juicing. There were not tons of options back then, so I drank carrot juice like crazy. It didn't matter—I was pouring healthy nutrients right into my bloodstream and I felt great.

- I cut out most processed foods.

- I cut out all processed sugar, including high fructose corn syrup, and raw cane sugar. Most important, I cut out all artificial sweeteners. These are cancer in a packet. Drop those things and never touch them again.

- I cut out all simple carbohydrates, such as cookies, cakes, pastries, white bread, and crackers. These items promote inflammation, creating the perfect, cozy home for cancer to grow.

- I cut back on my caffè lattes and reached for green tea instead.

- I cut back on my alcohol so I only had a glass of wine with dinner at a social gathering.

Here is what I wouldn't do again.

- I cut out all animal protein. At the time, the research I did showed a lot of benefits of a vegetarian diet. When I cut out animal protein, I felt lethargic and anemic. My energy was shot—not what you want while you are trying to beat cancer! When I added animal protein back in, I felt instantly better.

- I loaded up on dairy products. Since I had cut animal protein out, I used dairy as a protein source even though I knew it was not good for me. My body never handled cheese well and I had digestion and sinus issues that made that worse, but at the time I was totally lost about what to eat. Now, I know that there's always another option with nutrition and a little more research would have shown me how many beans, legumes, and veggies are protein-packed.

- I ate a lot of processed soy products with soy lecithin, soy protein concentrate, soy protein isolate, textured vegetable protein, or hydrolyzed vegetable protein, thinking they were good protein sources, instead of realizing they were just chemicals.

A vegetarian or vegan lifestyle isn't for everyone. As always, you need to listen to your gut and figure out what is right for you. I recommend keeping a food journal. Write down what you ate and how you felt. It sounds simple but the results will blow your mind. So many of my clients started noticing that their throat got itchy when they ate almonds or they got super gassy after eating eggplant. This sounds minor but it's your body's way of telling you it's rejecting those foods. And, yes, your body can reject healthy foods!

I don't do great with Brussels sprouts, tofu, or green peppers. David doesn't do great with beets, cilantro, or raw garlic. Pay attention to your body and it will give you the tools it needs.

Step Four: Kitchen Support

Convenience is the devil's playground. Think about the last time you were really hungry. Did your body say, "hey, why don't we swing by the farmers market and grab some produce, come home, chop it on up, and make ourselves a big salad?"

Doubt it! It probably said, "get me a muffin or a slice of pizza ASAP."

Our bodies are brilliant but they are still holding onto training from caveman days in which food was scarce. Now, we live in an overabundance of food and yet our body still is trying to get us to eat the thing that will quell our hunger quickest: sugar. When you're hungry, your body panics for you. It is literally screaming at you to eat cookies and donuts and that leftover pastry that you know won't be that good but it's available.

When my clients come to me and say they want to eat better, I tell them it's all about preparation. It takes a bit of work but it's the only way to long-lasting health.

I had an overweight client with stage 3 prostate cancer who lived alone. He had no clue about eating healthy and didn't know his way around the kitchen at all. I knew that I couldn't just give him an eating plan and hope he would follow it. So we started in his kitchen. We went through together and removed all the gluten, sugar, dairy, and processed foods. Well, now he had a fairly empty kitchen!

Next stop was the grocery store. His biggest concern was that he wasn't going to be able to afford the diet I was recommending. I educated him about how to eat healthy on a budget. We brought produce that was in season, frozen veggies that were out of season, and loaded up on inexpensive healthy meal fillers, such as beans, lentils, quinoa, and brown rice. He was not only surprised by how easy this was but he actually thought the food tasted better than what he had been eating.

After a few weeks of eating and shopping like this, weight started falling off him. His inflammation, swelling, and puffiness went way down so his joints didn't ache. He started sleeping without taking sleeping pills every night, and his energy and mood became better. His fight against cancer was completely turned around.

I know it's not always easy to prep healthy food and reach for celery when your body wants candy. But upping your preparation and decreasing your temptation will save you in the kitchen. I know for me, when I get hungry, I reach for potato chips. But guess what? If I don't buy them, I can't eat them. Simple as that. I try to load my fridge with cut veggies, hummus dips, coconut yogurt kefir, homemade protein bars, sprouted nut butters, quinoa salads, and green juices so I can never use convenience as an excuse. And don't fool yourself—there's no food faster than a fresh piece of fruit.

elissa goodman

Here is some advice I give my clients.

- Clear out the junk! Throw away anything with white flour, hydrogenated fats, trans fats, artificial chemicals, preservatives, fish contaminated with mercury, animal protein with hormones and/or antibiotics, GMO foods, fried foods, gluten, dairy, alcohol, and caffeine.

- Dairy is okay in moderation, but make sure you choose grass-fed options. I love grass-fed butter, ghee, feta, and goat cheese. Goat cheese is easier to digest than cow's milk cheese, so keep that in mind when choosing your dairy.

- Processed soy is a big no-no for me, but if your body can digest soy products, feel free to enjoy organic soy milk, edamame, organic non-processed tofu, and organic tempeh.

- Limit caffeine. I'd prefer you drink green tea, but if you love coffee too much to totally give it up—like me—then buy your own, organic, toxic-free beans, and brew your own coffee at home. Avoid coffee houses and limit yourself to one cup a day.

- Ideally, you cut out alcohol, but if you have it, moderation is key again. If your body can handle it, having a few drinks a week isn't the end of the world. Stressing about everything you consume can actually make you worse than if you just consume it. Sometimes people are surprised I'm okay with a little alcohol but sometimes that one glass of red wine provides you the relaxation and relief you need.

- Shop the outer limits of the supermarket, which is where whole foods are kept. Unless you are picking up beans, legumes, or whole grains, those inner aisles are just filled with tempting processed foods.

- Consume a rainbow. Eat a wide variety of veggies, fruits, nuts, seeds, and legumes. This ensures you are getting a wide variety of nutrients.

- Shop seasonally. This provides the freshest produce at the best prices.
- Shop your local farmers markets. This is the best place to find fresh and inexpensive produce. Talk to the people selling and ask them about their products. Often times, products are technically organic but it was too expensive for the farmer to pay for an organic license so the products aren't labeled as such. For those of you who don't have a local farmers market or aren't available to go when it happens, check online for community supported agriculture (CSA) boxes. This is an incredible and often inexpensive way to get a box of fresh, local produce delivered straight to your door.
- Be wary of pre-made juices that claim to be healthy. Fresh, raw, veggie juices with a small amount of fruit are best.
- Don't be afraid of fat! Moderately consume grass-fed butter, ghee, olive oil, coconut oil, nut and seed oils, nuts, seeds, and avocado.
- Explore other protein options. Legumes, beans, unprocessed soy, nuts, seeds, gluten-free grains, and certain veggies are a nice alternative to animal proteins.
- Animal protein should be unprocessed, without chemical additives or hormones. Meat should be from grass-fed animals and organic when possible. Animal foods should not be overcooked or burned.
- Eggs should be hormone-free, antibiotic-free, free-range, and organic when possible.
- Cut the sugar. Eat low-glycemic foods as sugar drives cancer cell growth.
- If you're craving something sweet, eat organic fresh fruit.
- Drink at least half of your body weight in ounces of water daily to flush unwanted toxins and chemicals from the body. If you can add fresh squeezed lemon, this would be amazing!

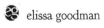

There are a million reasons to eat crap all day long. It tastes good, it's what the kids want for dinner, and you deserve it, that Pinterest recipe with all those low-fat ingredients makes you feel healthy. Trust me, I've heard and experienced them all. But there are a million and one reasons to make nutrition a priority—if you don't know the joy of cutting open the perfect avocado, if you want to have energy for the kids, if you think you deserve a long and healthy life, if you want to be glowing and radiating health and look your absolute best.

I promise if you do the steps above and make the effort to cleanse your kitchen, you will find that healthy food is fulfilling and satiating and delicious. Your taste buds, which are drowning under processed chemicals, will come back to you and you will know the true joy that food can bring. It's so easy to say we will start eating healthy Monday or next month, but I urge you to make it a habit and a lifestyle today.

In many ways this hack is the ultimate cancer hack. When you have a diagnosis, your world is turned upside down. We all deal with it in many different ways, but the need for a safe, calm cancer-fighting world is the same among us all. I did not write this book because I felt like I did everything right or because I am sure I know what you need. I wrote this book because I understand the importance of you figuring out what you need and going out there and getting it for yourself. We live our lives in default mode; we try to handle everything around us and take each moment at a time. So many of us worry about overwhelming others with our issues or taking up too much space or feeling too bold in what we ask for. This is your journey. This is your world. This is your environment. You control who comes in and out and you control what happens here. I want you to feel empowered to create a physical, emotional, and mental state in which your cancer starves and your spirit thrives. Why wouldn't you?

"I build a world around me that nourishes my body and soul, and I trust myself to make choices that help me thrive."

elissa goodman

Cancer Hacks: Closing

We've come a long way.

This book has been a huge journey for me. It is something I have thought about doing for years, but I never really thought I would do it. It has been scary, invigorating, and emotional to write this and I cannot believe I did it. When I beat cancer and found myself wanting to help others, I thought I would start with some friends, family, maybe a few friends of friends. As my business grew, and I was forced to acknowledge it as a legitimate business, each step was met with great trepidation.

Putting myself out there has been scary. My fears about not being good enough, not knowing what I was doing, not being able to help anyone resurfaced in a huge way. Writing this book has made me feel more exposed than ever. It has been such a personal and deep experience. I thought about things that I had avoided for years. I looked back at my life and really got to see the whole picture. When I was in it, everything felt like baby steps but when I look back, I see the leaps and bounds I have made.

My career began as a journey about nutrition, food, and supplements and then quickly turned into teaching me lessons about having faith in the universe. I can easily tell you what to eat or what supplements to take, but the most important thing I want you to understand is that you are in charge of your life and your healing. The purpose of this book is about regaining control over your health and mental wellbeing. It's about releasing your fears, facing the stuff that is scary, and recognizing how strong and powerful you are.

The medical world we live in today is scary. We all know people who have had or have passed away from cancer. It is a real threat. But getting a cancer diagnosis is not as scary as the medical community has made it out to be. Cancer doesn't need to be a death sentence. I see it as a wake-up call. Cancer is not telling you that the world has beat you down, it is the world asking you to stand up for yourself, stop underestimating yourself and your potential. It is telling you to get up and fight.

There is a reason you read this book. Whether you or a loved one has a cancer diagnosis or you're afraid of getting one, your interest in this book was most likely fear-induced. You are scared and you rightfully want answers. Living in fear is no way to live your life. I have spent many years of my life living in fear. I still sometimes do. It is a crippling place to be. But I have learned a lot about fear in the past few decades of my life. Fear is not the police officer you must obey; fear is the bully that puts up a tough exterior but will not resist once you fight back.

You can do this. You can take back your life. If I could take one thing away from you, it would not be you or your loved one's cancer. I would take away the fear. When cancer comes into your life, it is like a cold splash of water on your face. It is begging you to wake up. Something is wrong and only you have the power to fix it. There are so many options to help you heal and improve your life, but you have to be willing to take the first step.

When I am interviewed, people ask me what is one thing I would want their readers to know. I always say, I want them to know that if their life is making them unhappy or sick they have the power and the ability to change it. I always tell my clients, if you want this to happen, you can make it happen.

We get so caught up in being victims, feeling powerless, thinking that the things we want are unreachable or too hard or destined for someone else. I have watched it happen with my clients for years. I have no power over them, some see massive results, some don't. The difference has nothing to do with me, but it has everything to do with whether or not they really wanted things to be different. I am just a motivator and they are the elbow grease.

Sometimes people come to me and I can tell they do not want to be there and they do not really believe in what I do. But they came across my name and made an appointment and they are sitting in front of me. Something inside of them told them that maybe I had some answers for them. Maybe I could give them what they were looking for, even if they thought I was crazy. And maybe it was a small tiny flicker inside them, but they still heard it. And that is all that matters.

Are you paying attention? The entirety of my book can come down to four words:

Listen to your intuition.

All I could ever want is for people to reconnect with their instincts and their gut feelings and to understand that everybody already knows what they need. Everybody already possesses the tools they need to heal. No one else can tell you how to heal—not me, not your doctor, not your family, or your best friend.

Throw everything you know out the window and give yourself a chance to get to know you. Really take the time to find out if you are happy with your life, your relationships, and your work. I do not care what any doctor says in terms of percentages and numbers. This bugs the crap out of me! How would any doctor know what percentage of a chance you have to live? That is insane! Who you are on paper and your blood results are not your whole story.

Every time, I go to a Lakers game or a movie, I cannot help but eat the buttery popcorn. I know my stomach hates it and every time I feel sick afterward, but I still eat it. We have become a culture that still eats the popcorn every time, even though it makes us feel sick. We still go back to the job that makes us miserable, we still date the person who no longer makes us happy, we still hang out with the people who drive us crazy.

elissa goodman

We are taught that the good comes with the bad and some areas of our life just are not ever going to be perfect. When did we start accepting that?! We are so afraid of seeking out anything else that we pigeonhole ourselves into believing that everything is okay. You do not have to settle for any job, relationship, doctor, or disease. You do not have to settle for anything you do not want to settle for. It is important to tap into what is causing you to not get what you want out of life. I bet it is fear.

I did not do everything right when I got cancer. In fact, I did a lot of stuff wrong. If I had the chance to recreate my perfect plan for healing my cancer, it would be far different today. I had so many issues in my life to handle that I was only able to skim the surface of my own healing. The truth is, there is no perfect plan. Our life journeys are meant to play out exactly the way they do. We are usually where we are meant to be. I truly believe that I survived all my health issues and my cancer so that I could be here today to help you. I'm here to hopefully help save your life with some of my wisdom. If I can save a life, that is worth me recovering from cancer in itself.

You can never predict the outcome. There is nothing you can do to control your future. You cannot even predict how today will end. All you can do is control this exact moment right now and the choice you make right this minute. What happens in an hour, in a week, in a decade—that is not up to you right now.

So today, in this moment, what do you choose? Do you want to feel good about yourself? Do you want to seek happiness and healing? For most of you, the answer will be yes, but for some of you deep inside the answer might not be yes and that is okay. If you did answer a resounding yes and it came from deep inside your core, I hope this book will change and spark something within you to start fighting and healing. I want you to do everything you can to become the person you always thought you would be. I have all the confidence that you will find that person.

elissa goodman

When my clients have success with their physical and mental health issues, they come to me and tell me, "not only do I feel so much better, but I just got this great job offer or I finally fell in love, or I have a chance to move to Austin like I've always wanted to." This is not a coincidence. Without getting too crazy on you, you have to believe that there is something else working toward a higher good for your benefit and when you commit to taking care of yourself, you commit to finding happiness in all areas of your life. And if you are someone who doesn't believe in a higher power, that is okay too.

People fantasize about something or someone who makes them go to their cabinets and toss out the cookies, or pull the trash can up to fridge and wipe out everything, or make them sign up for a yoga membership, or start walking the few miles to work every day. We all want the life-changing moment where everything is just supposed to click and fall into place. You do not need these things to wake up. Maybe it is just the next time you are at the grocery store, you will buy more organic products. Maybe at work tomorrow you will check out the yoga studio downstairs. Maybe you commit to spending half your lunch hour going for a walk. I'm just asking you to take baby steps one moment at a time.

A friend of mine told me she had been wanting to try yoga for the longest time, but she wanted to do home yoga videos before she went to a class. I didn't understand this thinking. She said she didn't want to embarrass herself and she needed to maintain some sense of control. This felt like a lot of work to me that she needed to master yoga before actually taking a beginner's yoga class. We are constantly using excuses so we don't have to face our fears and insecurities.

If you want to stop letting fear run your life, then I would like to sign up to be your support. I truly believe in you. The answers might not seem obvious now, but they will come to you if you take it one day at a time. It is being more conscious of your choices, like grilled cheese or salad? TV or working out? Gratefulness or bitterness? Happiness or sadness? Fear or fearless?

elissa goodman

I am far from perfect. Some days I forget to eat lunch and eat a whole bag of potato chips instead. Some days I don't want to fight my kids on meatless Monday so I just make something I know they will like instead. I have skipped yoga for a drink with my girlfriends. I have picked *Game of Thrones* episodes over writing in my gratitude journal. I have said the wrong thing to my daughters. I have not been able to hide my frustration with my clients.

Some days it takes a team of people for me to get a blog post out and during the course of writing this book, you bet I have complained about having to sit down and write when I would rather be doing just about anything else. I should not be your role model or your hero. I am simply your cheerleader. I have been where you are. I have been exhausted, overworked, depressed, and overwhelmed. I still feel that way sometimes.

But most of the time now, I feel at peace and I feel a sense of calm. I feel in charge. I feel powerful and smart. I feel educated and in touch. This did not come easy or overnight. It has been a long path to understanding myself, my fears, and tuning into what my body was asking for all along.

I have learned to choose my battles. I do not get down on myself for being human. We are not meant to do everything according to some dumb plan. We are meant to fuel ourselves with good, and in turn we get good back. We are meant to do the best that we can every day. It is not the mistakes or the mishaps that will define us, it is our beliefs and how we ultimately live our life.

You are the most powerful force in your life. No one can take that from you. If you do one thing when you close this book, I ask you to start listening to YOU. What do *you* want? How do *you* feel? It's not about what worked for me or your friend, it's about what works for you. Everyone's journey is so different and we need to realize it.

So take a deep breath, clear your mind. Start asking yourself what you need to heal.

You have the answers. You have had the answers the whole time.

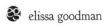 elissa goodman

Appendix 1

Protein Content of Selected Vegan Foods

The general rule of thumb for making sure you are getting enough protein per day is .36 grams per every pound of body weight. (If you weigh 150 pounds = 54 grams of protein intake per day.)

Soy

4 ozs. cooked tempeh	= 20 grams
4 ozs. cooked tofu	= 20 grams
1 cup cooked Edamame	= 17 grams
1 cup organic soy milk	= 9 grams

Beans/Legumes

1 cup cooked lentils	= 18 grams
1 cup cooked black, kidney, pinto, etc.	= 15 grams
1 cup cooked garbanzo beans	= 15 grams

Grains

1 cup cooked quinoa	= 9 grams
1 cup wild cooked rice	= 7 grams
1 cup buckwheat	= 6 grams
1 cup cooked oatmeal	= 6 grams
1 cup cooked millet	= 6 grams
1 cup cooked buckwheat = 6 grams	= 6 grams
1 cup cooked brown rice = 5 grams	= 5 grams

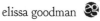

elissa goodman

Nuts/Seeds

2 tablespoons raw hemp seeds	= 10 grams
2 tablespoons raw pumpkin seeds	= 8 grams
2 tablespoons raw nut/seed butters	= 8 grams
2 tablespoons almonds	= 6 grams
2 tablespoons raw sunflower seeds	= 6 grams
2 tablespoons cashews	= 5 grams
2 tablespoons chia seeds	= 4 grams
2 tablespoons flax seeds	= 4 grams

Vegetables/Fruit

1 cup cooked green peas	= 9 grams
1 head romaine	= 8 grams
1 cup cooked/raw spinach	= 5 grams
1 tablespoons spirulina	= 4 grams
1 cup cooked collard greens	= 4 grams
1 cup cooked asparagus	= 4 grams
1 cup raw/cooked Brussels sprouts	= 4 grams
1 cup raw/cooked broccoli	= 4 grams
1 cup raw/cooked kale	= 3 grams
1 cup avocado	= 3 grams

Appendix 2
Guide to Eating Out
and in Restaurants

A lot of people say they want to eat healthier, but that they eat out too much to make it a realistic goal to achieve.

I want you to know that eating out can be healthy—you just need to know what to look for and what to avoid when you sit down to the table.

By following these tips, you can be confident that you are making the healthiest choices available without giving up your favorite restaurant!

- **Eat a small snack before you go out to eat:** A handful of nuts, ¼ of an avocado with sea salt, or a tablespoon of almond butter are all great options. Also, putting a couple teaspoons of chia seeds in 8 oz. of water will properly hydrate you and cut your appetite. Not arriving at your destination in a state of starvation will help you choose with a clear head

- **Pass on the bread basket:** If everyone at your table is in agreement about this, the best way to resist is to not have the bread in front of you. The waiter might be able to bring you some olives or cut-up veggies instead.

- **Start with a salad:** A lot of appetizers are fried or breaded, so sticking with a salad is a great way to have an appetizer course, but a much healthier one. For dressing, always ask for olive oil and vinegar or oil, lemon juice, and sea salt.

elissa goodman

- **Go for the protein and vegetables:** Grilled, roasted, or broiled fish, chicken, tofu, or lean meat, along with sautéed veggies are a safe bet. Ask if the chef can use olive oil and drizzle lemon on top. If you don't see any dishes prepared this simply on the menu, just ask. It's likely that the chef will be able to make it for you. Avoid sauces and dips, because they are laden with hidden sugars, poor oils, gluten, and dairy. Skip the starches and ask for double vegetables.

- **Know before you go:** If possible, check out the menu before you go, so that you can decide in advance what you'd like to eat. This way it won't be any trouble at all when you get to the restaurant because you will already have your plan in place. Many restaurants will note certain dietary restrictions, such as gluten and dairy free, on their menus. Additionally, some restaurants have a separate gluten-free menu that they will provide on request.

- **Suggest a healthy restaurant:** Are you able to choose the restaurant? If so, Clean Plates is a great restaurant guide, and picking your spot ensures you will have no trouble finding healthier eating choices.

- **Follow "hara hachi bu":** Do as the Okinawan Japanese do and stop eating when you are 80 percent full. Instead of eating until you are FULL, eat until you are NO LONGER HUNGRY!

- **Remember fruit is nature's candy:** Usually fresh fruit—especially berries that have a low glycemic load—is the best way to satisfy your sweet tooth. But, if you'd like to indulge a bit, share dessert with others at the table. You can satisfy your palate with a few bites and keep your body happy by not overdoing it. Another trick I like is BYO dessert! Stick a square or two of dark chocolate in your bag and have that instead of any dessert at the restaurant.

Appendix 3
Recommended Supplement
Brands and Resources

I have spent years curating the products, brands, and resources that I love. The market is always growing, but these are the products and experts I trust and rely on and turn to when my clients need some extra support.

Kitchen Products That I Like

Juicers—Breville JE98XL, Omega 68006

Blenders—Blendtec, Vitamix

Food Processor— Breville BFP800XL Sous Chef Food Processor or Cuisinart DFP-14BCN 14-Cup Food Processor, Brushed Stainless Steel

Cookware—Green Gourmet Hard Anodized Cookware by Cuisinart, Ecolution PFOA Free Water Based Non-Stick Hyrolon, Lodge Cast Iron

Supplements That I Like

Probiotics—Renew Life (a minimum of 50 billion beneficial bacteria); Enzymedica Pro-Bio; Dr. Ohhira's Regular Strength or Professional Strength

Digestive Supplements—Enzymedica Digest Gold ATPro

L-Glutamine—Pure Encapsulations; Jarrow; Natural Factors

Oregano Oil—Gaia

Grapefruit Seed Extract—Nutribiotic Liquid

Garlic Extract—Solaray Organic Odorless Garlic Capsules

Aloe Vera—George's Aloe Vera or Herbal Aloe Force

Black Walnut—Herb Pharma Certified Organic or Global Healing Center Paratrex

Wormwood—Herb Pharma Certified Organic or Global Healing Center Paratrex

Multivitamin—Certified Organic Synergy; Innate Response; Mega Food; Pure Encapsulations O.N.E. Multi (I take this one!)

OxyPowder (cleanse your bowels)—Global Healing Center

Spirulina—Nutrex Pure Hawaiian Powder or Capsules

Barley Juice Powder Extract—Vimergy

Zeolite—Omica Super Z Lite Liquid

Innate Response Innate Detox

Dr. Whitaker's Restful Night Essentials Extended Release

Magnesium Glycinate—Pure Encapsulations or Solaray

Ashwagandha—Organic India; Sun Potion; Wild Harvest

5-HTP—Pure Encapsulations or Jarrow

Kava—Gaia or Wild Harvest

GABA—Pure Encapsulations or Solgar

Other Products That I Like

Philosophie Protein Powders (vegan/Green Dream is my favorite flavor)

Flower Essence Services (FES) not Bach Flower Remedies

DoTERRA Essential Oils

Rosewater—Royal Sense Pure Bulgarian Rose Water

Mountain Valley Spring Water

Coconut Kefir Waters—Tonix or Healing Movement

Probiotic Drinks—Real Food Real Life

Kombucha—Synergy GTS or Health Aide

Coconut Yogurt Kefir—Tula's Coconut Yogurt Kefir

Sauerkraut—Sonoma Brinery

Kimchi—Rejuvenative Foods 100 percent Organic or Gold Mine Natural

Tempeh—Lightlife Foods

Flax Seeds—Spectrum Organic Cold Milled Premium or Navitas

Chia Seeds—Spectrum Organic Cold Milled Premium or Navitas

Hemp Seeds—Nutiva Organic Raw Shelled or Navitas

Websites That I Like

Environmental Working Group—www.EWG.org

A fabulous website that I use daily! Don't miss the many great consumer guides such as Shopper's Guide to Pesticides in Produce (updated yearly) and check the safety of your bathroom products in their Skin Deep database.

EWG has a cancer prevention site. They have compiled some of their best resources, blogs and new groundbreaking cancer research into one website aimed to inform and empower you with tips and tools to help stop cancer before it starts.

Seafood Watch—www.SeafoodWatch.org

Seafood can be so fishy! This site provides a guide to find and choose sustainable seafood in every state.

Mercola Skincare—http://www.mercolahealthyskin.com/products.aspx

Thrive Market—www.thrivemarket.com

Buy healthy food from top-selling, organic brands at wholesale prices. Shop for gluten-free, non-GMO, non-toxic products for a wide range of diets.

Vital Choice Seafood—www.vitalchoiceseafood.com

Vital Choice Seafood is your trusted source for the world's finest wild salmon and seafood.

Dr. Andrew Weil—www.DrWeil.com

Dr. Weil was one of my first mentors in this business and continues to be the godfather of the holistic health and wellness world. He is one of the smartest guys out there on these topics and I always utilize his website to stay up to date on new ideas and products. I always ask myself, "WWDWD: What would Dr. Weil do?"

FOODMATTERS | Daily Health and Wellness Inspiration—www.foodmatters.tv

Food Matters uncovers the secrets of natural health to help you achieve optimum wellness! Discover inspiring documentaries, wellness guides, nutrition tips, and more.

Dr. Nalini Chilkov Doctor of Oriental Medicine—www.nalinichilkov.com/the-healing-cancer-support-system.com

Dr. Nalini Chilkov, LAcOMD, combines her diverse training in traditional Oriental medicine, modern biomedicine and cell biology with 30 years in private practice. Dr. Chilkov primarily serves patients with cancer and complex, chronic illnesses alongside her optimal health and wellness practice. she is a respected expert in collaborative integrative cancer care known both for her meticulous attention to detail and individualized treatment plans as well as her warmth and compassion.

Mark Hyman MD—www.drhyman.com

Mark Adam Hyman is an American physician, scholar, and *New York Times* best-selling author. He is the founder and medical director of the UltraWellness Center and a columnist for the *Huffington Post*.

elissa goodman

Dr. Frank Lipman—www.drfranklipman.com

Founder and director of the Eleven Wellness Center in New York City, Dr. Lipman is a pioneer and internationally recognized expert in the fields of integrative and functional medicine. His personal brand of healing has helped thousands of people reclaim their vitality and recover their zest of life.

Dr. Axe—www.draxe.com

Dr. Axe is a certified nutrition specialist, expert in natural medicine, a speaker for Fortune 500 Companies (Nissan, Whole Foods) and a doctor of chiropractic.

Guided Light Healing—www.GuidedLightHealing.com

Alessandro Giannetti is an incredibly energy worker I have had the pleasure of working with in Los Angeles who truly performs healing miracles. If you are interested in energy work, be sure to check him out!

YogaGlo—www.yogaglo.com

My schedule is not always in-line with my yoga studio's schedule and YogaGlo has become a lifesaver for me! The site hosts online yoga classes at many levels that you can use whenever you want, wherever you are. Fabulous for traveling!

Calm App—www.calm.com

I don't let any of my clients leave without this app! This is a great introduction to meditation and even giving it five minutes a day will make you happier, calmer, and healthier.

Books That I Like

The China Study by Dr. T. Colin Campbell and Thomas M. Campbell

The Alchemist by Paul Coelho

Dying to Be Me by Anita Moorjani

Crazy Sexy Diet by Kris Carr

Mind over Medicine by Lissa Rankin, MD

You Can Heal Your Life by Louise Hay

Medical Medium by Anthony Williams

Radical Remission by Kelly A. Turner, PhD

Anticancer, A New Way of Life, New Edition by David Servan-Schreiber, MD, PhD

32 Ways to Outsmart Cancer: How to Create a Body Where Cancer Cannot Thrive by Dr. Nalini Chilkov

The 21 Day Sugar Detox: Bust Sugar and Carb Cravings Naturally by Diane Sanfilippo, BS, NC

Seeking the Heart of Wisdom by Jack Kornfield

Anatomy of the Spirit: The Seven Stages of Power and Healing by Caroline Myss, Ph.D

Cookbooks That I Like

Longevity Kitchen by Rebecca Katz and Mat Edelson

Nourishing Meals and the Whole Life Nutrition Cookbook by Alissa Segersten and Tom Malterre, MS, CN

Clean Food by Terry Walters

The Oh She Glows Cookbook: Over 100 Vegan Recipes to Glow from the Inside Out by Angela Liddon

How to Cook Everything: Completely Revised 10th Anniversary Edition by Mark Bittman

The Anti-Inflammation Cookbook: The Delicious Way to Reduce Inflammation and Stay Healthy by Amanda Haas

Cancer Fighting Kitchen by Rebecca Katz

True Foods Kitchen by Dr. Andrew Weil

Crazy Sexy Kitchen by Kris Carr

It's All Good by Gwyneth Paltrow

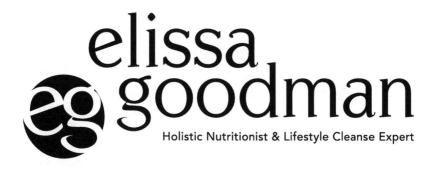

elissa goodman

Holistic Nutritionist & Lifestyle Cleanse Expert

7day

Healing Cleanse

Pre Cleanse Week

Let's talk about what this cleanse is meant to do for you. In our celebrity and perfection obsessed culture, cleansing has been mis-interpreted as a deprivation diet meant to shed weight fast. In this way, cleansing has become another form of yo-yo dieting and nothing about that is healing in any way.

This healing cleanse is beyond weight loss, beyond short-term goals, beyond vanity. To truly begin to heal, your relationship with your self and with your food must be redefined. This is a program meant to help you heal your relationship with food and your body. Your body is an intelligent, self-cleansing system, but in our modern world, we need to provide it with a little extra support sometimes.

You will feel more emotionally grounded, clearer minded, more energized, and in tune with your inner voice. The program will prepare your body to release toxins (microbes, parasites, metals, pesticides, to name a few). Most importantly, during these seven days, you will eat enzyme and nutrient rich foods that alkalize and decrease inflammation. You will support your detoxifying organs – lungs, skin, liver, kidneys, and colon – to help them operate better.

The benefit will go beyond surface level and will put you on a path to healing and that is my wish for you.

In order to prepare for your cleanse week, here are a few tips that will maximize your experience:

- **Choose a week that will work for you.** Look through your calendar and choose a week that you can really commit to preparing and cooking. This will take approximately 30 to 60 minutes each day. Read through all materials before you decide on your start date so you have realistic expectations of what the cleanse will entail.

- **The week prior, cut back on sugar, processed foods, gluten, dairy, and caffeine.** Cutting down on these gradually will ease you into the cleanse. To avoid headaches, irritability and other symptoms of withdrawal from caffeine and sugar, it is vital that you ease yourself off of them the week before.
- **Rest up! A cleanse requires a lot of internal energy.** The week prior to your cleanse, gear up by getting your sleep. See if you can go to bed earlier in 15-20 minute increments the week before, so each night you are getting more sleep.
- **Check in with yourself.** The week before your cleanse is a good time to outline and get in touch with your reasons for cleansing. It takes a deep purpose (beyond desiring a physical change) to commit and follow through with a cleanse. Take time this week to emotionally get in touch and discover why a cleanse will truly benefit you. What are you ready to let go of? Do you need more energy? Is the way you feel about yourself affecting your relationships? Have you had a health scare and need to make a change? Finding out what drives you will lead to lasting change.

elissa goodman

Your Cleanse Week

This program will not include any of the following inflammatory foods: processed foods, gluten, refined sugar, dairy, alcohol and animal protein. Don't panic! You will still enjoy and even love what you are eating. As your body heals and you become less chemically and emotionally addicted to these toxic foods, the cravings will dissolve.

You don't have to eat everything. Use this program to start practicing awareness about quality versus quantity in what you are eating.

If you feel full, do not feel pressured to finish any of the items. Your body is very likely adjusting to this new clean eating regime and is welcoming a break from the excess food.

Here are your cleanse tips for the week:

- **The Tools –** There is a lot of information here, but please take the time to read through it all. Read through all the recipes, too. None of the recipes call for any strange kitchen tools, but make sure you have what you will need. It's important that you do not feel caught off guard with any element of this process, so read through everything so you know what to expect. Preparation is your friend!
- **The Menu –** Included is a menu, schedule, and all your recipes for the week. You can follow the menu chart or substitute with another menu item from the same category. For example, if Day 4's salad doesn't sound appealing and you loved Day 1's salad, feel free to substitute. Also, your personal schedule might not allow for cooking every day so you can make double of any item to eat again the following day.

- **The Experience –** It is important for you to really experience this week. Do not choose to cleanse during a week in which you will be on and off the program. Give yourself the opportunity to dive in and really be focused on every aspect. Schedule time to cook and to eat. These items should not be hurried, stressful times. Do not make nourishing your body a rushed experience.
- **Substitutions –** You don't like sprouts? You have an issue with garlic or onions? Don't panic! Nothing will explode and be ruined if you skip these things. So long as you substitute with pure, organic, unprocessed foods, you will be okay!
- **Water and Lemon –** On this cleanse you will start each day off with water and lemon, but you are encouraged to drink water with lemon ALL day long! Lemon is highly detoxifying and a natural diuretic that will aid in flushing toxins out of your body. The combination of lemon and water loosens toxins held in your digestive tract. Lemon also purges toxins from your bloodstream, and combined with the hydration of water, the two make for a stronger immune system, more energy, and clearer skin!
- **Snacks –** If you feel hungry, first make sure you are drinking enough water. Dehydration loves to show itself in the form of hunger. If you are still hungry, there are optional protein based snack options included. Pick one to add in the afternoons when you are feeling hungry.
- **Animal Protein –** Some of us simply cannot go a week without animal protein, myself included. I limit animal protein when I cleanse, but abruptly transitioning to a vegan diet can induce weakness, exhaustion, and mental fog. If you find that you are eating the recommended amount of vegan protein and feel weak, tired, or mentally fatigued add in conscientiously raised animal protein such as turkey, chicken, lamb, fish, or an egg (organic, grass-fed, wild caught). Appropriate portion size is the size of your palm.

- **Protein with each meal** – Having plant protein with each meal or as part of a snack will stabilize your blood glucose levels. Think of your blood glucose as the fuel for your body. If you don't eat enough protein and your glucose levels drop, you impact not just energy, but your state of mind too! Low blood glucose levels correlate directly with low energy and irritability. In addition, when glucose levels drop, the body compensates by secreting cortisol from the adrenal glands, the center of our stress response, making it even harder to lose stub born weight! During your cleanse week, feel free to add plant protein to your soups, salads, and snacks. A list of suggested plant proteins supplements is included with your daily cleanse recipes.
- **Buy Sprouted Beans/Nuts/Legumes** – We are including these for protein options. If you have any problem with digesting them, please make sure to either buy sprouted or soak them for a minimum of 8 hours before cooking (make sure to throw out the water they soak in). This will allow for the outer phytic acid coating to be lessened and you will be able to digest and absorb their nutrients easier. We want to lessen any gas or bloating from happening this week! For even more convenience you can buy sprouted beans/nuts/legumes at your local health food grocer.
- **Eating Out/Picking Up Food** – Sometimes eating out is unavoidable. If that happens, choose a place that is organic, local and will offer some good vegan options for you. Follow your instincts and try to match what you order to what was planned for you. Keep it pure and simple. If you have a local juicer that you love and want to pick up your juices or smoothies- go for it. Use the recipes as a guide and try to match something similar, especially in terms of fruit-veggies ratio and make sure it is organic.

- **Coffee –** If you are a regular coffee drinker, going cold turkey isn't my recommendation. Having one cup per day with stevia or nut milk (optional), or switching to green tea in the morning, make cutting back more manageable. A little headache from your body adjusting to reduced caffeine is normal, be sure to drink lemon water and have a green tea if you need to power through.
- **Alcohol –** Sorry - you need to take a hiatus from the booze. While you are cleansing, it is a major no-no and actually counteracts the results of a cleanse. Even one drink can ruin your cleanse results instantly!
- **Exercise –** This program should not inhibit you from doing any of the exercise that you currently do. In fact, it is very important to get moving. Even just walking 30 minutes a day is amazing. Stick with low impact exercises like pilates, hiking and yoga.
- **Chewing Your Food –** It is very important to take the time to chew your food, because it is the first step to proper digestion. The way you chew, including how long you chew, can significantly impact your health in ways you likely never knew. Chewing your food thoroughly allows you to absorb more nutrients and energy from your food, maintain weight, keeps your teeth strong, reduces excess bacteria in your intestines and helps with digestive issues like gas and bloating.
- **Organic –** The produce you juice should always be organic. This stuff is going right to your cells, so you want it to be toxin-free! Organic products always have fewer pesticides and toxins, and are way less likely to be GMO. Take a look at the "Dirty Dozen" list of produce that you must buy organic and which items you have lenience with:
http://www.ewg.org/foodnews/summary.php

elissa goodman

- **Canned/Plastic Goods** – If you are buying any canned goods, please make sure they are in BPA-free cans. I prefer to buy the cardboard containers of items such as beans and diced tomatoes so I don't have to worry about the chemicals in the cans or plastic containers. Most plastic is super toxic. Again, anything you buy in a plastic container must be BPA-free. Most plastic water bottles are lined with carcinogens. Buy a glass or steel reusable bottle and carry it with you to avoid having to drink bottled water. Remember, a cleansed life is not just about the food. You have to be aware of environmental toxins too or you might as well not cleanse at all.

Post Cleanse Week

Congratulations on completing your healing cleanse week! You got through the ups and downs and have reset your system...doesn't it feel incredible? You have renewed your body and helped remove those cravings for sugar, processed foods, gluten, and dairy. You have probably noticed a difference in your complexion, your weight, and your energy. I assure you, the biggest difference is within a part of you that isn't visible to the eye. Now that you have completed seven days of eating clean, don't fall back into your old habits and addictions. Instead, feel motivated to live a cleansing lifestyle everyday, use this week as your guide…your journey to healing has only just begun!

Here are some tips to follow as you end your cleanse:

- **Eating Meat** – If you are a meat eater, make sure you are buying organic, grass-fed, hormone free animal proteins. Lean protein, such as organic free-range chicken and eggs or turkey, bison, and elk are great options. If you don't know where your meat came from, don't be afraid to ask. Follow a plant-based diet with meat a few days a week, instead of as the primary nutrient in your diet. Eating meat is a personal choice and having flexibility in your diet is perfectly okay, but the truth is meat is an inflammatory food and the more we can supplement with plant based foods, the less we are opening ourselves up to hormones, antibiotics, and inflammation!
- **Coffee** – If you must have coffee, try to have no more than one cup of organic coffee each morning and of course no cream or sugar. Sweeten with stevia if needed or add coconut, almond, or hemp milk. Coffee is dehydrating so if you do have coffee, up your water intake.

elissa goodman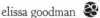

- **Dairy –** After seven days dairy free, your digestive system and skin have probably taken a turn for the better. Doesn't it feel good? This is a great time to explore plant based cheese and milk options in your diet. There are many on the market, including almond, cashew, and macadamia nut cheeses made with minimal processing.
- **Ease yourself into whole grains and gluten free options –** A week gluten free has shown you that it's very possible to live without pasta and bread! Now is a great time to explore quinoa, oats, buckwheat, farro, bulgar, lentils, and millet!
- **Continue with a juice a day –** You pack more nutrients and enzymes into your diet with a daily green juice. From a health standpoint green juice is great for your heart, your immune function, your digestive system, and in fighting cancer risks! If you take one thing away from your cleanse week, the importance of a green juice a day should be it!
- **Continue your lemon and water habit! –** Continue to start each day with lemon and water, this will not only aid digestion, but it will also help detox, fight cravings and boost your immune system.

Cleanse Menu & Schedule

DAY 1	DAY 2	DAY 3	DAY 4	DAY 5	DAY 6	DAY 7
8 oz. Warm Water with Lemon	8 oz. Warm Water with Lemon	8 oz. Warm Water with Lemon	8 oz. Warm Water with Lemon	8 oz. Warm Water with Lemon	8 oz. Warm Water with Lemon	8 oz. Warm Water with Lemon
Detox Tonic	Detox Tonic	Detox Tonic	Detox Tonic	Detox Tonic	Detox Tonic	Detox Tonic
Build Your own Juice or Smoothie	Build Your own Juice or Smoothie	Build Your own Juice or Smoothie	Build Y our own Juice or Smoothie	Build Your own Juice or Smoothie	Build Your own Juice or Smoothie	Build Your own Juice or Smoothie
Wild Rice Salad	Tahini Salad	Avocado Salad	Cauliflower Rice Salad	Faux Almond Tuna Salad	Brussels Sprouts Slaw with Hazelnuts	Must Have Make Ahead Salad
Broccoli and Arugula Soup w/ a side green salad	Creamy Curried Lentil Soup w/ a side green salad	Parsley and Pea Soup w/ a side green salad	Hearty Minestrone Soup w/ a side green salad	Carrot and Coriander Soup w/ a side green salad	Cauliflower, White Bean, and Rosemary Soup w/ a side green salad	Caribbean Black Bean Soup w/ a side green salad
Tulsi or Herbal Tea	Tulsi or Herbal Tea	Tulsi or Herbal Tea	Tulsi or Herbal Tea	Tulsi or Herbal Tea	Tulsi or Herbal Tea	Tulsi or Herbal Tea

* During your cleanse week add plant protein to your soups, salads, and snacks. To calculate the recommended daily protein for your body weight, multiply .36 grams by your body weight. If you are extremely active, multiply your body weight by .5 grams (example: 150 pound individual should eat a minimum of 54 grams of protein daily, while an extremely active 150 pound individual should eat a minimum of 75 grams of protein daily).

* Keep Herbamare, a blend of salt and herbs (found at Whole Foods or online) on hand to spruce up any salad, soup, etc.

elissa goodman

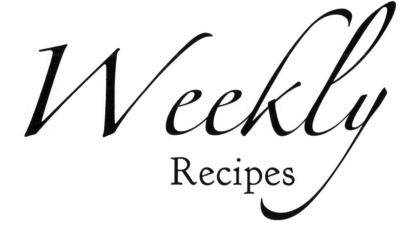

Weekly
Recipes

Start your day with warm water with lemon, followed closely by my detox tonic. Then a few hours later have a green juice or smoothie. You are giving your body a big burst of nutrients and your digestion a well needed break.

Detox Tonic
Serves 1

Ingredients:
2-4 ozs. coconut kefir (I use Tonix or Healing Movement)
2-4 ozs. aloe vera (I use George's Aloe Vera)
1-2 tsp. Bragg's apple cider vinegar
Juice of ½ a lemon
2 inches fresh ginger, juiced
6-8 ozs. water or coconut water
Optional addition: 1/8 tsp. cayenne and/or turmeric
(can also use high quality powder)

Directions:
Mix all ingredients together, and served chilled

Build Your Own Green Juice or Smoothie
Serves 1

Ingredients:
Start with 2 cups dark leafy greens (kale, spinach, parsley, arugula, romaine, dandelion greens, collards, beet greens, ect)

- **Add any of the following vegetables:** cucumber, celery, broccoli stems, carrots, beets, fennel, asparagus
- **Pick one low-glycemic fruit:** lemon, lime, apple, pear, tangerine, grapefruit, orange, kiwi, banana (smoothie only), berries (smoothie only), ¼ avocado (smoothie only)
- **Add some spice:** fresh ginger root, cinnamon, turmeric, cayenne, fresh parsley, fresh cilantro, fresh basil, fresh mint
- **Add healthy fats and Omega 3's:** 1 T. of cold-milled flax seeds, 1 T. chia seeds, 1 T. hemp seeds, 1 T. Bulletproof XCT Oil, or 1 T. organic coconut oil (the medium chain fatty acids are sent directly to the liver where they are immediately converted into energy. It will actually speed up your metabolism too)
- **Add plant based boosters:** Amazing Grass Raw Reserve, Navitas Gelatinized Maca Powder, E3 Live (blue green algae), Nutrex Hawaiian Spirulina, Vimergy Barley Juice Extract Powder
- **Add plant-based protein (smoothies only):** Sun Warrior Vegan Protein, Philosophie Green Dream Protein Powder, Nutiva Hemp Protein Powder, or Health Force Warrior Natural Vegan Protein
- **If you need sweetener (optional):** Omica Organics Liquid Stevia or Body Ecology Stevia

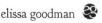

elissa goodman

Tulsi or Herbal Tea
Serves 1

Ingredients:
8-10 oz. water
1 bag Tulsi or decaf herbal tea (chamomile, peppermint, dandelion, ginseng, licorice root, ginger)*

Optional: 100% pure stevia, organic unsweetened hemp, almond, or cashew milk

*If you are having any problems with constipation, I suggest Traditional Medicinal's Smooth Move Tea

Vegan Protein Options to Supplement Meals

Soy
4 ozs. cooked tempeh = 20 grams
4 ozs. cooked tofu = 20 grams
1 cup cooked Edamame = 17 grams
1 cup organic soy milk = 9 grams

Beans/Legumes
1 cup cooked lentils = 18 grams
1 cup cooked black, kidney, pinto, etc. = 15 grams
1 cup cooked garbanzo beans = 15 grams

Grains
1 cup cooked quinoa = 9 grams
1 cup wild cooked rice = 7 grams
1 cup cooked millet = 6 grams
1 cup cooked buckwheat = 6 grams
1 cup cooked brown rice = 5 grams

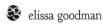 elissa goodman

Nuts/Seeds
2 tablespoons raw hemp seeds = 10 grams
2 tablespoons raw pumpkin seeds = 8 grams
2 tablespoons raw nut/seed butters = 8 grams
2 tablespoons almonds = 6 grams
2 tablespoons raw sunflower seeds = 6 grams
2 tablespoons cashews = 5 grams
2 tablespoons chia seeds = 4 grams
2 tablespoons flax seeds = 4 grams

Vegetables/Fruit
1 cup cooked green peas = 9 grams
1 head romaine = 8 grams
1 cup cooked/raw spinach = 5 grams
1 tablespoons spirulina = 4 grams
1 cup cooked collard greens = 4 grams
1 cup cooked asparagus = 4 grams
1 cup raw/cooked brussels sprouts = 4 grams
1 cup raw/cooked broccoli = 4 grams
1 cup raw/cooked kale = 3 grams
1 cup avocado = 3 grams

* During your cleanse week add plant protein to your soups, salads, and snacks. To calculate the recommended daily protein for your body weight, multiply .36 grams by your body weight. If you are extremely active, multiply your body weight by .5 grams (example: 150 pound individual should eat a minimum of 54 grams of protein daily, while an extremely active 150 pound individual should eat a minimum of 75 grams of protein daily).

Approved Snacks and Juices

Snacks:
- Flax or rice crackers with 2 T. organic raw almond butter
- Raw veggies of your choice with ½ cup organic hummus
- Flax or rice crackers with ½ smashed avocado sprinkled with hemp seeds
- 12-15 sprouted almonds, pumpkin seeds, walnuts, or cashews
- ½ cup edamame tossed with 1/4 avocado, diced
- 1 super seed bar (see recipe)

Beverages:
- Ultima Replenisher Hydrating Powder (Whole Foods or online)
- Fresh raw organic coconut water
- Plain 100% organic kombucha
- Add in an additional green juice
- Chia Lemonade - 16 ozs. filtered water, 1 T. chia seeds, fresh squeezed lemon or lime, stevia (optional)
- Tulsi Tea

Super Seed Bars
Makes 12 Bars

Ingredients:
1 ½ cups gluten free rolled oats
1 ¼ cups brown rice crisp cereal
¼ cup hemp seeds
¼ cup sunflower seeds
¼ cup unsweetened shredded coconut
2 T. sesame seeds
2 T. chia seeds
½ tsp. ground cinnamon
¼ tsp. fine grain sea salt
½ cup Coconut Secret Coconut Nectar
¼ cup organic almond butter
2 tsp. organic vanilla extract
¼ cup goji berries, cacao chips, or pumpkin seeds (could also use nuts of your choice)

Directions:
Line a 9-inch square cake pan with two pieces of parchment paper (one going each direction)

In a large mixing bowl combine the oats, rice cereal, hemp seeds, sunflower seeds, shredded coconut, sesame seeds, chia seeds, cinnamon, 1 teaspoon vanilla and mix well.

In a small saucepan, stir together the coconut nectar and almond butter until well combined. Cook over medium to high heat until the mixture softens and bubbles slightly, then remove the pan from the heat and stir in 1 tsp vanilla.

Pour the nut butter mixture over the oat mixture, using a spatula to scrape every last bit out of the pan. Stir well large

elissa goodman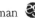

spoon, until all of the oats and cereal are coated in the wet mixture (the resulting mixture will be thick and slightly hard to stir). If you use the cacao chips, allow to cool slightly before folding in the chips, if you use goji berries, you can add anytime.

Transfer the mix to the pan prepared with wax paper. Spreading it into an even layer, lightly wet your hands and press down on the mixture to even it out. Use a roller to compact the mixture firmly and evenly. This helps the bars hold together better. Press down the edges with your fingers to even out the mixture.

Place the pan in the freezer, uncovered, and chill for 20 minutes, or until firm. Lift the oat square out of the pan, using the parchment paper as handles, and place it on a cutting board. Using sharp knife, slice the square into 6 rows, then slice in half to make 12 bars total. Wrap bars individually for best storage.

Keep in airtight container in fridge for up to 2 weeks or you can store extra in freezer for up to a month.

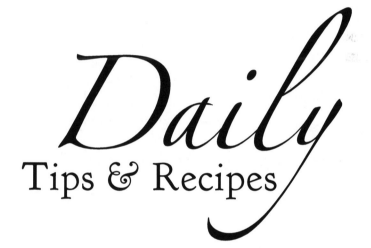

Daily

Tips & Recipes

Day 1 Tips & Recipes

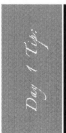

Lemon water, lemon water, lemon water. Staying hydrated is key during your cleanse week. We are made up of 55%-70% water! Water intake supports us on a cellular level and drinking just any old liquid won't do! Herbal tea, vegetable juice, and fruit juices can count towards your daily water tally, but coffee, tea, soda, anything containing alcohol do not count as water intake and actually dehydrate the body!

As you cleanse, you will be flushing toxins from your body and staying hydrated supports your body in doing so. As a rule, throughout your cleanse week (and every day!), you should consume a minimum of half your body weight, in ounces, per day.

That means, a 150 pound female should drink a minimum of 75 ounces (Approximately 9 glasses) of water per day.

Why is staying hydrated vital? Proper fluid balance:

- Supports brain function
- Fights fatigue and is a natural energy source
- Curbs hunger, since thirst is often mistaken for hunger pains, staying hydrated will curb "hunger"
  and support metabolic functioning
- Flushes kidneys and rids the body of waste material
  and toxins
- Promotes digestive health
- Provides a healthy glow and good skin
- Transports nutrients and oxygen to cells

Wild Rice & Butternut Squash Salad with Maple Chili Tempeh

Serves 4

Ingredients:
1 cup wild rice blend, uncooked
½ tsp. sea salt
2 T. organic olive oil
2 cups butternut squash, diced
2 T. coconut oil
8 oz package of LightLife Tempeh
1 T. maple syrup
2 T. tamari or coconut aminos
½ tsp. chili powder
¼ cup dried or fresh blueberries
⅓ cup pecans, toasted and chopped
Juice and zest of 1 lemon
Juice and zest of 1 orange
½ cup parsley, fresh chopped
Sea salt and pepper

Directions:
Preheat oven to 400 degrees. Line a baking sheet with parchment paper. Add wild rice blend to a pot and cook according to directions (add salt). Toss the butternut squash in the olive oil, sprinkle with salt. Arrange in a single layer on the baking sheet. Bake for 20-25 minutes, until fork tender but not mushy. Set aside.

While squash cooks and rice steams, cook the tempeh. Cut into 1 inch cubes. Heat coconut oil in sautee pan and medium high heat. Place tempeh in the hot oil in a single layer and cook for until golden and crisp on each side (approx. 1-2 minutes per side). Add the maple syrup, tamari, and chili mix to the sauté pan and toss to coat the tempeh.

elissa goodman

In a large bowl, fold the cooked rice, butternut squash, maple coated tempeh, pecans, and blueberries. In a bowl, whisk the maple syrup, chili powder, and tamari together. Add the lemon juice & zest and the orange juice & zest. Add salt and pepper as needed and garnish with fresh parsley.

Broccoli and Arugula Soup
Serves 4

Ingredients:
2 T. olive or coconut oil
1-2 clove garlic, thinly sliced
½ yellow onion, roughly diced
1 medium organic Yukon gold potato, peeled and diced
1 large head broccoli, cut into small florets (about 2/3 pound)
5 cups water or vegetable stock
1 cup arugula (can also use watercress)
½ lemon, sliced
Salt and pepper to taste

Directions:
Heat the oil in a nonstick saucepan over medium heat. Add the garlic and onion and sauté for just a minute or until fragrant. Add the potatoes and broccoli and cook for four minutes, stirring often, until broccoli is bright green. Add the vegetable stock, Herbamare and pepper, and bring to a boil, lower the heat and cover and cook for eight minutes or until the broccoli and potatoes are just tender.

Carefully pour the soup into a blender and puree with the arugula (or watercress) until quite smooth. Start slowly and work in batches if necessary (you don't want the steam to blow the lid off).

Serve the soup with a squeeze of fresh lemon and season with additional salt and pepper if needed.

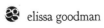 elissa goodman

Day 2 Tips & Recipes

Consider a diet free of sugar, gluten, dairy and processed foods. The challenge of these foods is that they are addictive on a cellular level. Our cells don't know how to totally digest these staples of the mainstream American diet. Our cells metabolize some nutrients, but get stuck with a lot of remnant waste. That remnant waste clogs our cellular intelligence and our bodies start to crave what they already have: junk!

This cleanse will aid you in combatting your cellular addictions. You will rid yourselves of that clingy junk once and for all by flushing your body with waste clearing daily juices. You can conquer cravings by eating really nutrient rich, life-promoting foods.

Here are a few things to consider in regards to gluten, sugar, and dairy:

- Gluten causes gut inflammation in at least 80% of the population and another 30% of the population develops antibodies against gluten proteins in the gut. Gluten's inflammatory effect in the gut causes intestinal cells to die prematurely and causes oxidation on those cells. An unhealthy gut means that food is not being digested properly and nutrients are not being absorbed fully, which can lead to nutrient deficiencies.
- Sugar has been strongly associated with cancer. In addition sugar is inflammatory, contributes to lower immune system functioning and increased cellular aging.
- We're the only species (other than those we are domesticating) that drinks milk after infancy. And, we're definitely the only ones drinking the milk of a different species. Not only are the naturally-present hormones in cow's milk stronger than human hormones, the animals are routinely given steroids and other hormones to plump them up and increase milk production. These hormones can

elissa goodman

negatively impact humans' delicate hormonal balance. Commercial feed for cows contain all sorts of bad ingredients, including: GMO corn, GMO soy, animal products, chicken manure, cottonseed, pesticides and antibiotics. Yuck!!

Tahini Salad

Serves 2

Ingredients:

2 cups romaine, shredded
¾ cup red quinoa, cooked
¼ cup carrots, diced
¼ cup red cabbage, shredded
¼ cup kalamata olives, pitted
1 T. organic tahini
1 cup garbanzo beans, cooked
1 clove garlic

Directions:

Blend tahini, lemon juice, garlic, sea salt and pepper in a blender until well combined. Add filtered water as desired until you reach your desired consistency. Combine all other ingredients and drizzle with dressing.

Creamy Curried Lentil Soup
Serves 4

Ingredients:
3 T. organic coconut oil
1 large yellow onion, chopped
3 medium stalks organic celery, chopped
2 large carrots, chopped
2 large cloves garlic, chopped
1 inch fresh ginger, grated
2 ½ T. yellow curry powder
1 T. sea salt or Herbamare seasoning
½ tsp. cayenne powder
1 bay leaf
1 cup dried red lentils
3 cups water (for soaking lentils)
4 cups organic vegetable or chicken stock
16 ozs. organic full fat coconut milk

Optional garnish: cilantro, diced green onion, pepitas, pumpkin seed oil

Directions:
Soak the dried lentils over night in 3 cups of water, add a squeeze of lemon. This will help in digestion and absorption of the nutrients (you can use un-soaked or sprouted lentils if preferred).

Prepare the onion, celery, carrot, garlic, and ginger and set aside. Heat coconut oil in a large soup pan or stockpot over medium high heat. Once heated, add the chopped vegetables, sea salt or herbamare, garlic and ginger and stir continuously over medium heat for 8-10 minutes to prevent garlic from burning and to allow vegetables to soften.

Once vegetables are softened and onions are translucent, add the curry powder, cayenne,and bay leaf. Stir well and saute for another 2-3 minutes to blend the flavors. Add the strained lentils and vegetable or chicken stock (making sure lentils are covered by the stock, if needed add more).

Allow soup to simmer for 15-20 minutes on medium low. When lentils are softened, add the coconut milk and stir well. Very carefully add the cooked soup mixture into a high-powered blender or Vitamix. Blend well, until soup is pureed and creamy. Add back to pot and serve warm.

You can garnish with cilantro, pepitas, or pumpkinn seed oil.

Day 3 Tips & Recipes

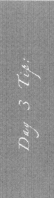

Supplement with a daily probiotic. Total well-being starts in the gut! Probiotics promote a healthy gut and clear our system of bad bacteria, while keeping the good. Probiotics can ease digestion, control sugar cravings, support a strong immune system, and will help you lose weight.

Everyone should be taking a strong probiotic daily, as that is the best way to get your gut in check. In addition to a 50-100 B strand probiotic supplement, you can also get major doses of probiotics from your food. But please don't eat those sugar-packed "probiotic" yogurts they won't do you any good!

Here are some healthy, probiotic-rich foods that you can add into your daily regimen:

- **Coconut Water Kefir –** This fermented beverage is made from coconut water, and contains both lactobacillus and bifidobacteria, which help create good intestinal flora, that will help you digest food easier and utilize B vitamins in your system. Coconut kefir hydrates and cleanses the intestines and liver and contains the same vitamins, minerals, and electrolytes as coconut water. My two favorite brands of Coconut Water Kefir are Tonix and Healing Movement
- **Coconut Kefir Yogurt –** Starting your day with this probiotic yogurt is an easy way to add probiotics to your diet. Made with organic coconut meat, coconut kefir, and a probiotic capsule, this yogurt is easy to make at home and store for the week. Recipe can be found at www.elissagoodman.com or you can purchase Tula's Coconut Yogurt.
- **Sauerkraut –** Sauerkraut is probiotic-loaded food and a good source of B vitamins. If you are scared of eating sauerkraut because you fear the not-so-sexy side effects a healthy dose of cabbage can leave behind, sauerkraut is

elissa goodman

easier on the system to digest and won't leave you feeling so gassy. A favorite fermented sauerkraut option is Sonoma Brinery.

- **Tempeh** – Fermented whole soybean is made by culturing and a controlled fermentation process. It has a firm texture and earthy flavor and can take on many flavors. Tempeh has the same protein quality as meat and contains high levels of B5, B6, B3, and B2.

- **Miso** – Miso is a really special probiotic food because it has a super low pH which allows it to get deep into the stomach and bypass the acidity. It also works to create B vitamins and vitamin K, flooding your system with nutrients and goodness.

- **Kimchi** – Kimchi is an unbelievably amazing probiotic superfood and a great side dish to virtually any dish. It contains probiotics that will do wonders on your gastrointestinal system as well as boost your immunity.

- **Kombucha** – Kombucha is full of amino acids, probiotics, antioxidants, healthy enzymes and loads of vitamins and other nutrients. One caveat- it can be a little hard on the system. Start with a few ounces daily and work your way up to only 8 ounces per day. Some people dive right into a 16 oz. bottle and feel sick and therefore never have it again.

Avocado Salad
Serves 2

Ingredients:
4 cups head romaine lettuce, torn into bite-size pieces
2 T. hemp hearts
1 small cucumber, diced
2 T. fresh mint, chopped
½ red bell pepper, diced
2 T. fresh parsley, chopped
1 large avocado, diced
2 T. cilantro, chopped
¼ cup pumpkin seeds toasted

Avocado Dressing:
3 T. water
2 green onions, chopped
3 T. lemon, freshly juiced
1 clove garlic, chopped
4 T. organic extra virgin olive oil
½ tsp. sea salt
pinch pepper
1 avocado, halved and fesh scooped out

Directions:
Put all ingredients in a blender and blend until smooth. Seasonal with additional salt if needed.

Toss the lettuce, cucumber, and bell pepper in a bowl. Drizzle with the dressing and toss again. Add the avocado, hemp hearts, pumpkin seeds, mint, and cilantro and toss once more.

Reserve additional dressing and keep in refrigerator up to 3 days.

elissa goodman

Parsley and Pea Soup
Serves 4

Ingredients:
1 T. coconut oil
2 medium onions
4 cloves garlic
1 lb. shelled green peas (frozen is fine)
2 cups parsley, leaves only
5 cups organic vegetable broth
1 lemon
1 T. extra virgin olive oil
Salt and pepper to taste

Directions:
Roughly chop onions and mince garlic.

In a large stock pot, heat coconut oil. When melted, add onions and a couple pinches of salt, stir to coat and cook for 5-10 minutes until onions have browned. Add garlic, stir to coat, cook three minutes.

Add 3 cups veggie broth, add peas, bring to a simmer and turn off the heat. Add parsley and fold in until it wilts. Transfer to a blender and blend on high until smooth. Add extra broth if desired.

Zest lemon and add to soup. Juice lemon and add to soup with olive oil, blend. Season to taste.

Pour back into the pot and heat through. Serve.

Day 4 Tips & Recipes

Raw foods, juicing and greens are important to detoxing, but nothing is as crucial during your cleanse week as rest. During your cleanse week, prioritize 9 hours of sleep EVERY night for the best benefit!

Here are some important factoids on the benefits of catching some zzz's during your cleanse week:

- Melatonin, the sleep hormone and a major antioxidant in our body is produced when you sleep. Shortening this output puts you at risk for a lot of major diseases. The colors of sunset actually trigger your body's production of melatonin-nature is signaling your body to rest. You need to listen to it!
- Just one night of bad sleep will raise your cortisol levels and set your hormonal levels off course, causing your body to hold on to excess fat!
- Your body clock resets itself between the hours of 10pm and 2am. Getting to sleep at 10pm is ideal for optimal cellular renewal. Aim to get to bed by 10pm during your cleanse week!
- Sleep promotes your body's production of antioxidants, your natural killer cells keeping your immune system strong.

Cauliflower Rice Salad
Serves 2

Ingredients:
½ head of cauliflower, leaves removed and chopped
½ cup snap peas, roughly chopped
½ cup radishes, sliced1 handful cherry tomatoes, sliced in half
¼ cup fresh parsley, roughly chopped
¼ cup fresh mint, roughly chopped
¼ cup roasted pumpkin seeds
¼ cup organic extra virgin olive oil
1 fresh squeezed lemon
Salt and pepper to taste

Directions:
Pulse cauliflower in food processor with slicer blade attached until it resembles rice. Spoon into a bowl.

Add all other ingredients except pumpkin seeds and mix well. Adjust seasonings as needed. Add more oil, lemon and/or salt and pepper if desired.

Sprinkle with pumpkin seeds and serve.

Hearty Minestrone Soup
Serves 6

Ingredients:
2 T. olive oil
1 medium onion, diced
2 stalks of celery, diced
1 carrot, peeled and diced
2 cloves garlic, minced
14 ozs. diced tomatoes with juice
½ cup fresh parsley, chopped
4 cups organic vegetable stock + more to taste
2 zucchini, diced
1 cup green beans, chopped
2 cups cooked cannellini beans
2 cups spinach, roughly chopped
½ cup basil, roughly chopped
1 tsp. dried oregano
1 tsp. dried thyme
Sea salt and pepper to taste

Directions:
Heat olive oil over medium heat in a soup pot. Add onion and pinch of sea salt and cook 2-3 minutes. Add carrots and celery and cook another 2-3 minutes. Add garlic and cook until vegetables are softened.

Add tomatoes and juice, parsley and pinch of salt and cook, stirring for a few minutes. Add the stock and a pinch of sea salt, oregano and thyme and simmer 1-2 minutes. Add the green beans and let simmer for a few minutes. Add zucchini and let cook for another 10 minutes, until soft.

Add more vegetable stock if needed. Add the cannellini beans, spinach and basil and heat through. Adjust seasonings as needed and serve. Add vinegar, basil and spinach and cook until heated through.

elissa goodman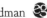

Day 5 Tips & Recipes

Day 5 Tip: Healthy fats are good for you. Fat has a bad reputation, but good fats, like olive oil, walnut oil, pumpkin seed oil, coconut oil, nuts/seeds, chia/flax seeds, avocado, etc. are actually crucial to good health and for weight loss. In particular, Omega 3 fatty acids are amazing for your body and are necessary for everyday processes the body has to go through. Omega 3's work to cut cravings for carbs and sugar, keep you full longer and will boost your vitamin and minerals.

Healthy fats:

- Have antibacterial, antifunfugal, anti-parasite and antiviral properties to help prevent illness
- Make you exquisitely attractive, they are essential in the absorption of many beauty vitamins and minerals, especially fat-soluble vitamins like A, D, E and K. They keep the hair shiny and your skin supple
- Provide excellent antioxidants supporting immune health

By the time you are done with these seven days, your body will be begging for some more pure, clean, healthy fats!

You can reconsider how you view fat in your diet and start by making these changes:

- **Eliminate trans fats from your diet as much as possible.** Check food labels for trans fats. Eliminating fast foods, premade baked goods, fried foods, and processed snack foods are some of the easiest ways to reduce trans fats consumption.
- **Know your good fats.** Don't be afraid of using ghee, organic coconut oil, organic extra virgin olive oil, pumpkin seed oil, nut butters, walnut oil, avocado, wild salmon, nuts and seeds.

- **Limit your intake of saturated fats with a plant-based diet, limiting red meat intake.** Try switching from dairy milk to plant based milks like almond, hemp, and coconut.
- **Eat omega-3 fats or take a daily supplement to boost intake.** Good sources include fish, walnuts, almonds, sesame seeds, sunflower seeds, pumpkin seeds, ground flax seeds, flax seed oil, hemp seeds, and chia seeds.

Faux Almond Tuna Salad
Serves 2

Ingredients:
1 cup raw almonds, soaked
2 celery stalks finely chopped
2 green onions, finely chopped
1 garlic clove minced
3 T. vegan mayo (suggested soy free veganaise)
1 tsp. Dijon mustard
½ fresh squeezed lemon juice to taste
Pinch of kelp granules (optional)
Salt and pepper to taste
1 English cucumber (peeled if desired) and sliced into 1cm rounds

Directions:
Soak almonds in a bowl of water for 3-9 hours until plump. Drain and rinse well. Add almonds into a food processor and process until finely chopped. It should look a bit like flaked tuna. Place into a medium mixing bowl.

Add the chopped celery, green onion, garlic, mayo, mustard, and lemon into the bowl. Stir well to combine. Season to taste with salt and pepper. Add a pinch of kelp granules if desired.

Slice cucumber into rounds, if using. With a small spoon, gently scoop out the center of each cucumber round to create a small well. Spoon

elissa goodman

the almond mixture onto each cucumber round. You can also serve it on gluten free cracker or on top of greens. Refrigerate leftover salad for up to 3 days.

Carrot and Coriander Soup
Serves 4

Ingredients:
2 T. olive oil
1 onion, chopped
2 cloves garlic, crushed
1 tsp. fresh thyme
1 T. ground coriander
6 very large carrots
½ cup fresh parsley, chopped (or about 8 medium carrots), peeled and chopped
5 cups vegetable stock
Salt and pepper to taste
Bunch of fresh cilantro, chopped

Directions:
Heat the oil in a large pot, then add the onion, garlic, and thyme, and coriander and sauté until soft. Add the carrots, parsley, and salt and stir-fry for 2-3 minutes. Pour in the vegetable stock, bring to a boil, then cover the pot and simmer for about 45 minutes, until the carrots are tender.

Remove from the heat and allow to cool, then puree until smooth. If the consistency is too thick add more vegetable stock and puree. Adjust seasonings to taste and heat through before serving. Sprinkle with cilantro and serve.

Day 6 Tips & Recipes

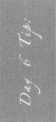

Day 6 Tip: Start each day with an affirmation! Flooding your body with nutrient-dense foods is amazing, but flooding your being with positive thoughts is beyond powerful. When you daily affirm yourself, you ignite the spiritual side of cleansing. With positive affirmations, you feel wonderful in body, mind and soul!

You can use the affirmations sent to you daily to build self-esteem, curb your impulse cravings and remind yourself of your intention! Here are some supportive affirmations that you may choose to use during your cleanse week and beyond as you take this journey to well-being.

- I lovingly do everything I can to assist my body in maintaining perfect health.
- I am ready. I am ready for a new body. I am ready for….
- I lovingly forgive and release all of the past. I choose to fill my life with joy. I love and approve of myself.
- I am at peace with my own feelings. I am safe where I am. I create my own security. I love and approve of myself.
- I choose and enjoy healthy, nutritious foods. I pay attention to my body and provide it with what it craves.

elissa goodman

Brussels Sprouts Slaw with Hazelnuts and Dates
Serves 2

Ingredients:
⅓ lb. brussels sprouts, shaved
¼ cup unsalted, raw hazelnuts, chopped
½ cup chopped pitted dates
2 T. extra virgin olive oil
2 T. apple cider vinegar
½ T. raw honey
¼ tsp. salt
cracked pepper to taste
zest of one orange

Directions:
Finely slice brussels sprouts or process in food processer with slicing blade attachment in. Place in a bowl, added chopped dates and hazelnuts.

In a small bowl, whisk together olive oil, vinegar, honey, salt and pepper. Pour dressing over slaw. Mix in orange zest and mix well. Adjust seasonings as needed.

Cauliflower, White Bean, and Rosemary Soup
Serves 4

Ingredients:
2 T. organic olive oil
1 T. Herbamare
½ T. sea salt
1 cups white onion, chopped
2 cloves garlic, chopped
2 bay leaves
2–3 sprigs rosemary, chopped
1.5 lbs. organic cauliflower, broken down
1– 6 ozs. box white beans, soaked and cooked
5-6 cups organic vegetable stock
pinch black pepper

Directions:
Add olive oil to soup pan and heat over medium high. Add salt and Herbamare, onion and garlic with 2 bay leaves. Sweat for 5-7 minutes, stir often. Add rosemary, continue to sauté for additional 2-3 minutes, stirring often. Add cauliflower and sauté a couple of minutes then add beans and vegetable broth. Bring to low rolling boil.

Simmer for 20 minutes (until cauliflower is fork tender, but not mushy). Add black or white pepper. Blend until velvety smooth.

elissa goodman

Day 7 Tips & Recipes

Daily de-stress. Finding ways to decrease stress and relax essential on this cleanse and in living a cleansing lifestyle. Stress promotes production of cortisol and can have the following impact on your life:

· It can make you hold on to fat around your middle section.
· It raises your blood sugar, creating sugar cravings.
· It depresses your immune system.
· It can damage your gut and lead to problems with food intolerances.
· It can cause infertility
· It can worsen PMS.
· It can accelerate aging.
· It makes you more likely to have cognitive decline
· If you gain weight, your cortisol levels will go even higher.
· It can make you depressed- 50% of people with depression have high cortisol levels.

Here are some easy ways to relax and lower cortisol production:

- Meditating in the morning is a great way to set your self up for a strong, stress free day. An easy way to start is by downloading calm.com on your mobile phone or computer
- Exercise, like a brisk 20-minute afternoon walk or 45 minute yoga session, is also an excellent way to increase happiness and decompress.
- Take a nightly detox bath (hot water, 1 cup Epsom salts, 2 cups Baking Soda, few drops of lavender essential oil and soak for 30 minutes to let your muscles soak in the goodness.
- Turn off your electronics 2-3 hours before bedtime. Make your bedroom a computer and cell phone free zone. The liberation feels phenomenal!

Must-Have Make Ahead Salad
Serves 4

Ingredients:
2 organic beets, peeled and grated
4 stalks organic celery, thinly chopped
1 organic English cucumber, thinly chopped
3 T. organic olive oil
3 T. organic fresh squeezed lemon juice
Himalayan sea salt and freshly ground black pepper
1 organic avocado, diced
5 T. raw sprouted sunflower seeds
3 cups organic wild arugula

Directions:
In a large bowl, mix beets, celery and cucumber. Add avocado, sunflower seeds, olive oil, lemon and salt and pepper and gently toss. To serve, spoon mixture over bed of arugula.

elissa goodman

Caribbean Black Bean Soup
Serves 4-6

Ingredients:
2 T. organic coconut oil
1 white onion, finely diced
5 organic roma tomatoes, chopped
2 jalapenos, finely diced (de-seeded)
1 tsp. Herbamare seasoning
½ tsp. cumin
4 cups cooked black beans, rinsed and drained
4-5 cups organic vegetable stock
½ bunch organic cilantro, chopped
Sea salt (if needed)
½ cup SO DELICIOUS culinary coconut milk

Directions:
Heat 1 T coconut oil over medium heat in a soup pot. Add onion, tomato, salt.and jalapeno and sautee until softened, approx. 4-5 minutes. Stir well. Add black beans, vegetable stock, and cilantro. Simmer on low for 15 minutes.

Carefully scoop the soup into a blender. Add coconut milk and blend until smooth. Pour this mixture back in to the soup pot and simmer on low.

Season with additional salt or Herbamare if needed.

Congratulations,
you did amazing!

I would love for you to share your experience with me

https://www.facebook.com/elissa.goodman.holistic.nutritionist

https://twitter.com/ElissaGoodman

http://instagram.com/elissagoodman

http://elissagoodman.com

About Elissa Goodman

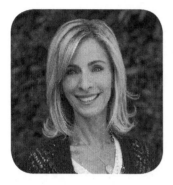

Elissa Goodman is a holistic nutritionist and lifestyle cleanse expert who believes that proper nourishment and a daily renewal practice are essential for optimal living. Through a journey of healing herself from Hodgkin's Lymphoma at age 32, losing her husband, and raising two beautiful daughters, Elissa has found that balance, nutrition and self-love are the best medicine. Elissa's mission is to educate and encourage healthy, mindful living helping others embrace the concept that we are a product of what we eat and how we treat ourselves. Creator of "Cleanse Your Body, Cleanse Your Life" and "S.O.U.P. Cleanse, her approach is gentle and accessible for those looking to renew, recharge, rejuvenate and maintain their healthy lifestyle. She is based in Los Angeles and works privately with professionals and celebrity clients to develop personalized wellness programs that encourage true health from the inside out. Specializing in a unique blend of conventional and holistic nutrition, Elissa includes supplement and superfood recommendations in her approach and supports clients with a range of health goals including those working to reset their metabolism, overcome auto-immune, digestive and inflammatory challenges or heal themselves from disease. Elissa creates a partnership with each of her clients teaching them to become their own health advocates and guiding them tap into their personal instincts. Results of her work are above and beyond learning to nourish yourself properly, lose weight or look good as she teaches you how to heal your gut and how to listen to it, encouraging clients to thrive. Elissa collaborates with health

elissa goodman

and wellness partners throughout Los Angeles and is the creator of M Café's macrobiotic RESET Cleanse, signature juice blends at Erewhon Market and L.A. Juice, and multiple recipes soon to be found at Earth Bar. She is a Certified Integrative Nutritionist from the American University of Complementary Medicine for Integrative Nutrition and holds a BS in Advertising & Marketing from Arizona State and BS in Business from the University of Arizona.

For more information, visit **www.elissagoodman.com**.

Made in the USA
San Bernardino, CA
28 September 2016